TIRED & TESTED

Sophie McCartney

TIRED & TESTED

The Wild Ride into Parenthood

Harper North

HarperNorth
111 Piccadilly,
Manchester, M1 2HY

A division of
HarperCollins*Publishers*
1 London Bridge Street
London SE1 9GF

www.harpercollins.co.uk

HarperCollins*Publishers*
1st Floor, Watermarque Building, Ringsend Road
Dublin 4, Ireland

First published by HarperNorth in 2022

1 3 5 7 9 10 8 6 4 2

A catalogue record for this book
is available from the British Library

HB ISBN: 978-0-00-847529-1
TPB ISBN: 978-0-00-854234-4

Printed and bound in the UK using 100%
renewable electricity at CPI Group (UK) Ltd

FSC
www.fsc.org
MIX
Paper from
responsible sources
FSC™ C007454

This book is produced from independently certified FSC™ paper
to ensure responsible forest management.

For more information visit: www.harpercollins.co.uk/green

For Jack & Evelyn,
Thank you for affording me two of life's greatest privileges:
becoming a Mummy … and being able to legitimately
use a 'parent & child' parking space.

Contents

Introduction

Welcome to the Jungle

There's something I've recently come to realise about parenthood, and that is you will never be ready. Much like the arrival into adulthood, no entrance exam is required, no instruction manual distributed, and there's absolutely no way of knowing if you're doing it properly.

The responsibility takes even the most mentally prepared by surprise, sneaking up from behind like a ravenous predator intent on devouring your freedom, figure, finances, and faff. One minute you're young, carefree, and busting shapes on a dance floor. Then, in the blink of an eye, you're mid-thirties, unable to remember your name but able to recite *The Gruffalo* as though it's the Lord's Prayer, and crying over a busted pelvic floor. The journey from perky tits to killing nits has well and truly begun.

How did you get here and, more importantly, where did you go? Although technically an 'adult', because I've trained myself to eat olives, most days I feel more like an out-of-depth teen trapped in the slightly saggy skin-suit of a 37-year-old tired and tested mother of two. An invisible bearer of snacks, who sidelines as a living napkin, the new life I've found myself living resembles nothing of what came before. My evolution from non-maternal to hu*mum*kind is an excellent example of Expectation vs Reality: life is not as initially anticipated. I have no idea what I'm doing, if the 'five-second rule' applies to houmous or whether my questionable parenting techniques will produce well-rounded individuals or future serial killers. One thing I know for sure is that, like most parentfolk, I 100 per cent have NOT 'got this' – unless, of course, we're referring to parasitic organisms.

If you've picked up this book hoping for parenting advice, toilet-training tips and homework hacks, you may be sorely disappointed … just like the visitors to Center Parcs' Subtropical Swimming Paradise after my child shat in the wave pool. Think of this more as a safe space of collective fuck-ups, life lessons, and discoveries that'll hopefully make you feel a tiny bit better about your own abilities – or life choices.

Whether you're pre-kids, in the eye of the baby storm or would rather choose pets over people, even the thought of responsibility for another living being can be mind-bending. When it comes to entering into the terrifying thought process of making and raising humans, if you didn't laugh, you'd cry … while rocking in a corner and questioning whether the brown stuff under your fingernail is Play-Doh, or something left over from a traumatising family staycation. It's an adventure, and one many of us wouldn't swap for the world (but definitely for half an hour), so sit back, grab a lukewarm cup of coffee, strap yourself in and join me as we head off on the wild ride into parenthood …

1

In the Beginning

… there was nothing. No stretch marks, no saggy boobs that flap like a spaniel's ears on a windy day, and no prior knowledge of the pressure a perineal massage can put not only on a rectum but on a marriage.

To set out my stall and truly take you on my personal voyage into the occasionally overwhelming realm of adulthood, first we need to go on a *Bill & Ted's Excellent Adventure* back in time to when low-rise jeans are responsible for a high rise in fanny flashing, and 90 per cent of the female population has FINALLY grown out the shortest layers of their 'Rachel' cut.

Welcome to the glory decade of the noughties! The year 2002 BC (Before Children) to be precise – a golden era of over-plucked eyebrows, jaunty trucker hats, and puking WKD Blue all over your mum – *Exorcist*-style – while pretending to have food poisoning. Things are simple here … face fillers are just what you get if you give the wrong person a dirty look in your local Wetherspoons; we're yet to question the size of our arses or lips;

and the dark, shapeshifting art of contouring is yet to be discovered. It's not that appearance isn't important in the stone-washed age of Juicy Tubes – I mean, if your white frosted eyeshadow doesn't shimmer like a frozen dog shit on a winter's morning, and you don't have upwards of seven belts attached to a minuscule denim miniskirt, are you even a real *Cosmo* girl? It's the calm before the selfie/social media storm and thanks to cameras and phones still being two separate and brick-like entities, there will sadly be very little future evidence of how well we slay these iconic looks. An utter travesty.

In this brave new post-Spice Girls world, 18-year-old me is spotty, unworldly, awkward, and semi-convinced that if I could *just* get myself to LA then I might still stand a chance with Leonardo DiCaprio. It's a great age, though, isn't it? Absolutely brimming with giddy anticipation, beautiful yet dangerous naivety, and a truly terrifying misguided sense of invincibility. 'Nothing's going to get me, bitches – I survived platform trainers and Sun In!' Up until this point, I've spent most of my life in Liverpool – a city famous for history, football, and arguably the greatest musical talent of our time … Atomic Kitten. But times are a-changing for this not overly academic, all-girls Church of England high-school leaver. With a set of A level results reading like a glamour model's bra size, I'm flying the nest and heading north of the wall to the jewel in Yorkshire's crown: Leeds. Here, I plan to drink all the brightly coloured alcopops my gag reflex can handle and blow my student loan on irresponsible non-curricular activities. Oh, and study Public Relations – not 'Pubic Relations' as my dad initially feared (but which is totally top of the extra credit priority list).

Yes, REAL LIFE BOYS! A very exciting prospect to someone whose only real relationship experience (aside from imaginary ones with Hollywood actors) is with a guy who, prior to dating, I first stalked from behind a bus stop for 18 months. Not entirely convinced a predatory, slightly obsessive infatuation was the best foundation for our courtship, he joined the air force fairly soon after we (officially) met, completely lost his loving feeling, and ruthlessly ejected me from the relationship. I cried for fourteen days straight, while listening to Alanis Morissette and slagging him off to all my mates on MSN. He, however, would not BRB.

It's not that I'm even mad keen on the prospect of settling down into anything long term, let alone getting married. Relationships are for old and boring people, not 18-year-old-girls with student loan 'free' dough and wild oats to sow. No, truth be told, I'm quite looking forward to getting out there and putting all the knowledge I've gleaned from *More!* magazine's highly ambitious 'Position of the Fortnight' to good use. How hard could a nice and gentle 360-degree 'Passion Propellor' be? All that's required is a greasy, inexperienced teenage boy flailing around on top of you like a malfunctioning Chinook, and boom! Welcome to womanhood! Tell you what would be a better column for the impressionable youngsters reading these magazines: 'Position of the Foreskin' – it might just help with the initial shock of seeing a penis in a turtleneck.

Despite puberty for me somehow bypassing breast development, opting instead to give me thick black lustrous armpit hair (Mother Nature? More like Brother Nature – no woman would do that to her own), I'm optimistic the next few years of university will provide a multitude of morality-testing opportunities – all of which will stick two fingers up to my religious education, despite my shit tits and yeti pits. There will be drinking, debauchery, dickstractions – and in these confusing times when I ask myself, 'what would Jesus do?' I'm fairly positive he'd respond with 'Pubic Relations'.

One thing, for sure, that's not going to happen to me at university (or at any point in the immediate future) is to become embroiled in a relationship with a highly immature, codependent, emotionally unstable individual. No, not a member of the undergraduate rugby team … but a baby. NO THANK YOU. Not today, Satan! Why would I? Being in your late teens/early twenties is a once-in-a-lifetime 'the world's your oyster' opportunity, and I'm all for being totally shellfish. No responsibilities, no commitments, zero baggage, all the sleep in the world, and all you have to do is steer clear of STIs (Stupid Tattoo Inscriptions) and not get knocked up – if that's not yet on your 'to do' or, more aptly, 'who to do' list. It's certainly not on mine. In fact, teenage me has a pathological fear of babies, small children, and basically anyone under the age of 16. Therapising myself here … my phobia more than likely stems firstly from being the youngest in my family – I've just never been exposed to the (literal) shit that comes with having younger siblings. And secondly, Chucky.

On seeing babies, rather than thinking 'I can't wait', my first thought is 'why are they here?' Shortly followed by, 'where's their kitchen knife?' What do they want from us? I'm not entirely convinced it's love, because all they seem to do is scream at their keepers, which seems really rather quite unreasonable given a lot of them enter the world as vaginal battering rams. They don't seem particularly happy to be here either. Very angry at everyone and everything for no particular reason – like mini members of UKIP, which is ironic because once you have them you never kip again. They have very clammy hands too, with sock fluff in between their fingers. SOCK FLUFF! Surely that should be in between their teeny tiny toes – which I'm also scared of, yet simultaneously want to eat and I DON'T KNOW WHY. At what point in Brother Nature's grand plan did he programme women – predominately – to want to eat small chubby children like they're Mini Rolls? Man logic! 'Let's give her cannibalistic tendencies – seems like a safe trait to have around young children, and might make her more inclined to give blow jobs.

Win-win!' He's basically gone and created small humans in the image of man after too many alcoholic drinks – a bunch of legless, ravenous, irate, boob-obsessed, urine-covered piss-takers.

Their vulnerability is also absolutely petrifying. Babies definitely don't seem like the kind of creature I'd be capable of looking after. Head control is an issue too. When I was about eight, I held my baby cousin for the first time and – I kid you not – his skull near-on rolled off his body as though he'd just popped four pills and was about to have a singalong to 'Wonderwall'. I thought I'd broken him! I can't even describe the panic. You know that feeling when you drop a mug at someone's house? It was like that, but with the additional fear of prison time. In the thousands of years humans have been in existence, why have we not evolved to do more from an early age? Did you know humans are one of the only animals that are defenceless from birth? We as a species are completely dependent on our parents until we're 30. Doesn't happen in the wild, does it? You don't see lion parents trying to leave the Pride Lands weighed down by four different change bags and a six-pack of fromage frais. *'Fuck's sake, Simba, hurry up! The hyenas are after the cubs! How do you STILL not know how to unfold the pram?! Not so much of a mighty king now, are you?!'*

And the thought of one living inside me and its subsequent eviction is also an incredibly off-putting prospect. Apparently, the pain is similar to period pain ... if you happen to be menstruating at the same time as being savagely attacked by a shark. At 18, as someone who struggles to insert a 'heavy flow' Tampax, I just can't get my head around the fact my vagina allegedly has the expandable properties of Mary Poppins' carpetbag – enough space for an actual human being, and a freestanding floor lamp. Forget a spoonful of sugar, I'm going to need a spoonful of crack cocaine. And how do you even find someone you like enough to consider procreating with? Presumably it starts with a search for someone with the small shoulders and hip circumference of an Olympic gymnast. It's a minefield, and to be honest, I'm not sure I want to walk across it unprotected.

If I decide on marriage, will I be a good wife to someone? Probably not. If babies eventually come for me, will I be a good mother? Absolutely not. I'm scatty, selfish, disorganised and an eternal time-optimist – I can hardly look after myself, never mind a child. The last life I was responsible for, other than my own, now resides, slowly starving to death and occasionally mewing for help, somewhere deep within the bowels of my bedside table. How can I be entrusted with the youth of tomorrow, if I can't even look after a bloody Tamagotchi …?

There's a lot this newly independent young woman wants to do with her life, such as travelling the world and having eye-opening, culturally stimulating, soul-searching, life-altering experiences that will enrich my body and mind … *Oi Ayia Napa, Ayia Napa, Ayia Napa, Oi!* Sun, sea … and vomiting blue curacao from my nose, all while falling in love with holiday reps who give away free shots but never their cold, cold hearts.

I want to live my life to the full, for it to be fully mine – answer to no one and go where I want to go, when I want, and all at the drop of a hat. Even though I don't know the finer details of what I want to *be* when I'm a proper, real-life grown-up, I want success, power, and to pay for things with my own (overdraft's) money. *Oh, the shoes on my feet? HSBC bought them!* There needs to be possibilities, fun, adventure, and a life less ordinary. These wild oats are not ready to be milled down into Ready Brek dust. I'm terrified at the prospect of giving up my womb, figure, career (that I don't have yet) and boobs (that I also don't have yet) – it all seems so sacrificial. I understand the theory behind having children – so the favour of arse wiping can be returned in later life – but I cannot and will not become a boring, married, kitten-heel wearer who's unable to drink more than two glasses of wine without pole dancing with a lamp post. Nor will I turn into a knackered, screamy shell of my former self, a herder of children who lives in houmous-covered stretchy trousers and occasionally leaks from various orifices. No. I will go as far as CATEGORICALLY saying that I will never, ever become one of *those* tired and tested women …

2

Beaver Fever

Whitney was curious as to how she'd know. Phil's mum told him not to hurry – that he'd just have to wait, and Bono scaled city walls like a UV-ray-averse Spider-Man and he still couldn't find what he was looking for. Which begs the question, how do you go about finding 'the one'? And if you want children at some point in the future, what makes the perfect mating partner (slender bone structure aside)? By my twenties, I was massively struggling to find someone I could tolerate long enough to share chips and dip with – never mind gametes. For some, it's as easy as lust at first sight ... for others, it's more disgust. Regardless of how you get there, for a lot of us, the journey to happily-ever-after can feel like a very long and grinding road ...

When it comes to relationship expectations, I personally feel as though we have a lot to blame Hollywood for – not poor Paul, although I do gain two stone every time *Bake Off* is on. No, as in

Tinseltown – home to glitz, glamour, egg-white omelettes, and movies filled with unrealistic expectations. Unknowingly, us gals have been drip-fed a constant churn of unachievable, unhealthy, and unacceptable bullshit for years. Everyone knows the only decent way to eat yolk-less eggs is in a meringue. Animals.

Looking back, I realise the silver screen planted so many ridiculous romantic ideologies in my head, making my teenage years and meeting the likes of a boy locally referred to as the 'Kappa King' (pubes on his top lip and shitfaced on Hooch) down at the youth-club disco all the more disappointing. In that dingy church hall, there was no Patrick Swayze dance teacher and inappropriate student sexual relations, no 'gu-gums' or 'baby in the corner' … well for me anyway, but I'm pretty sure that's how it ended for one of the Year 11 girls. No, the closest I got to 'dirty dancing' was accidentally grazing the semi-flacid sceptre of polyester royalty while energetically flinging my body-glittered arms around to 'Cotton Eye Joe'. Where did it come from? Where did it go? And why was it such a shock? Static from all the synthetic fibres, I imagine.

Late-teen me was NOT overly desperate for serious, long-term commitment – the ones we meet first are very rarely the ones who take us up the aisle; they may take us up other places, but it's highly doubtful a vicar or your nan would be there watching. They are for practice only because, of course, practice makes perfect … fun. When all the oats have been sown however, what then? Obviously, I eventually wanted to find someone who loved me unrequitedly – who wouldn't? Someone to be my equal, to unwaveringly support my questionable life choices, and who'd take the bins out. Yes, even if in the short term I ended up dropping blokes faster than Elizabeth Taylor shed husbands, long term, finding 'the one' was actually of great importance to me. The question, however, remained: how do you go about hunting them down?

Contrary to what Phoebe from *Friends* led us all to believe, lobsters don't actually mate for life; they're monogamous for about two weeks and then fuck off to pastures new and seaweed green – presumably under the guise of being on a break. It's the beavers we want. They're committed little bastards – they find a soulmate with equally shit teeth, similar enthusiasms for wood-based DIY and then they never let go. They are totally happy with their lot and have zero desire to look elsewhere seven years into the relationship. No, you never get an itchy beaver.

So how do we all become more 'giant rodent' in our approach to finding love? Well, the first hurdle to overcome is relinquishing those misguided delusions of snogging the likes of Channing Tatum in the rain, Kevin Costner guarding your body, or being so irresistible to a 300-year-old hunky vampire that the minute you shag him he loses his tortured soul and tries to eat your mates. It's pretty hard to establish a normal relationship capable of living up to those expectations. I spent many a year expecting to find the love of my life as a result of a tense, high-speed hostage situation on the number 86 bus into Liverpool, courtesy of a maniacal retired bomb squad officer. Thanks, Keanu. Funnily enough, I only ever found a weirdo with his hands down his pants fiddling with an entirely different type of explosive device.

Our infatuation with finding romance and being rescued, in my opinion, starts quite early on in our lives, stemming from everyone's favourite magic kingdom ... not IKEA, but Disney. I now look back on so many of my favourite childhood 'classics' with serious questions about how they may have skewed my perceptions of female ambition, and the place of women in relationship dynamics. I mean, Ariel gave up her voice to enable a man to fall in love with her for Christ's sake! The most horrifying part, retrospectively, is that the only concerns six-year-old me had about that film were centred around the logistics of having a mermaid tail and needing a poo. How did she go? Did she want to be part of the human world so badly because of severe constipation? Snow White kicked it all off, though, back in 1938, didn't she? Not only was she rescued by handsome royalty, but he also brought her back to life with the power of one kiss. Talk about raising the bar! Now, thanks to her, many of us pine for a hero with a snog so powerful it functions as a defibrillator (although a vibrator might be more useful …). Then it was Cinderella's turn – kick-starting the female infatuation with crippling heels and the notion that a 'glow-up' makeover, combined with a cute dress, could solve all our worldly problems. Her one-night stand bagged her not a venereal disease, as we've all been warned, but actual Prince Charming and the best castle on the 'Far Far Away with the Fairies' block. She might have been a stunner, but the woman thought she could talk to birds, made outfits for mice, and probably smelt like piss and biscuits. Meanwhile, Aurora, aka Sleeping Beauty, taught us love conquers all, including the small matter of a bloke breaking into your home and taking advantage of you while you're unconscious. Then there was Belle, paving the way for classic 'saviour syndrome', though to be fair to her, the beast was a grade-A HUNK – but only in animal form (controversial, I know). My fear here is that she unwittingly encouraged many a female to dedicate years of their lives trying to change brooding beefcakes with anger issues and a penchant for incarceration. You say Stockholm, I say Syndrome.

Thankfully, for most of us, life doesn't turn out like a Disney film – otherwise a lot of children would be orphaned by the time they turned five. Wouldn't you just love to see where those princesses are now, and how their relationships are going? Did they really get their 'happily ever after' or has Snow reverted back to her wild-child days of living with multiple male partners? Has Prince Charming, highly impulsive with an unhealthy foot fetish, eloped with a crying drunk girl he found outside a chicken shop looking for her shoe? Is Cinders now in the grip of a mental collapse, covered in bird shit and singing to pigeons in Central Park? My biggest hope is that Aurora's now fully wide awake and has ditched Prince Phillip to become the poster child of the Once Upon a Time 'Me Too' movement, main objective … rescuing Belle from the dungeons after a misjudged waxing suggestion of a back, sack and crack.

When it comes to the rocky path of finding true love, it seems that the charade of finding 'the one' is actually much more difficult than we've all been led to believe by misinformation and movie directors. Will we ever be rewarded with heart-stopping smooches, a handsome yet troubled stripper, or princely perfection? Well, some of us do instantly, others … we must first kiss a few beavers.

Dating nowadays, for Gen Z especially, appears to be quite different to that of my old-school millennial dating days. So much has changed, and I can't decide whether it's easier or harder on the other side of Y2K. One thing's for sure, though, kids today will never know our struggle of trying to be in a relationship with someone we couldn't internet stalk first. Combine that with risking life and limb every Saturday night ironing our own hair, and it's a bloody miracle we all survived to tell the grim(m) fairy tale. Yes, what a bunch of lucky fashionable bastards these newbies are with their *Teen Vogue* good looks and 200°C of GHD ceramic smoothing power at their fingertips. What did we have? Our mums' Morphy Richards Steam Plus, which just removed our fingertips. We were smoking hot … literally. There was no Tinder, Bumble, or Plenty of Catfish, either. No, if we wanted to find our knight in shining Ben Sherman, we had to go out into the battlefields of Yates's, Oceania, Liquid, Inferno (insert your own sticky-floored, STI-riddled local club here), for it was there our blue-shirt-wearing, greasy-haired dreamboats were waiting, ready to sweep us off our feet with killer pick-up lines like 'nice tits'.

After such romantic wooing, there would follow the mating ritual of shit dancing, a sloppy snog and a drunken fumble before exchanging numbers on your mobile brick. After waiting the obligatory two days to text them back, and a few Pizza Hut all-you-can-eat buffets later, you were in dangerous Lynx Africa Christmas-present-buying territory. Now, there's this whole unspoken process that has to happen for a certain level of commitment to be reached. I know this after a huge amount of extensive, highly academic research into the subject – otherwise known as *Love Island*. For under-rock dwellers unfamiliar with this, it's a reality TV programme in which the physically beautiful put their lives and hearts on the line for the whole world to see, in a hopelessly romantic bid to find their true … social media following. From what I've observed, this is my basic understanding of how the new-fangled and fickle courting process works. First, the approach – normally as a result of one party sliding into the other's DMs (personally my younger self would have gone mad if someone I didn't know wore my Dr. Martens, but we're living in a different time, so each to their own). Next, a bit of 'flanter', which I believe is the term for 'flirty banter' and not the name of a carbonated orange beverage, followed by some 'sexting', which, with more than 160 characters to play with and a whole host of innuendo emojis, is much more of a provocative event than it was in the technological dark ages of the early noughties. (.) (.)

Chaps are also getting to grips with a completely different 'snake' to that of the Nokia 3210 days, with many opting to use the rapidly evolving advancements of telecommunications for the power of … dick pics. Lads, funnily enough, an unsolicited picture of a button mushroom skewed to the spikes of a hedgehog carcass doesn't have us sliding off our chairs with excitement.

I think I speak for many women when I say this, but make better choices – lighting, positions, filters – 'Paris' the shit out of that penis. Next, if their cock-tail sausage hasn't caused long-term damage to the retinas of the receiver, a hook-up may ensue. It could be for drinks, or a bonk in a bush, but the most important thing to remember is that it remains SUPER casual. Only after ten or more of these meets are you allowed to progress to the next round … dating. Totally noncommittal, it's very much akin to the probation period when you start a new job – it gives everyone a kind of get-out-of-jail-free card. Shock horror – this phase isn't straightforward either and there are several variables to consider, such as how Instagrammable said person is, DMs from other potential suitors, and something called 'fanny flutters', which I think is a trendy name for thrush. Once, and only once, you have safely moved past this level, you can FINALLY declare yourselves … exclusive. Which is apparently NOT the same as being boyfriend and girlfriend/girlfriend and girlfriend/boyfriend and boyfriend, and allows you to shag someone else without being classified as a dirty cheating lobster. Congrats! Yes, the path to 'making it official' is as long as it is painful, and when the time comes to pop the 'big question' and commit to that serious relationship, I imagine most people say yes because they're about to draw their pension and haven't got any other options.

Thankfully, my exploration into the world of relationships happened several years in advance of the dating equivalent of *The Hunger Games*. Sadly, it didn't mean the odds were ever in my favour. My boyfriend stat sheet read like a knock-off series of *Friends* – 'The One with the Girlfriend', 'The One with the Erectile Issue', 'The One with a Dolphin Laugh', 'The One with the Weird Belly Button', 'The One Who Got Naked in Public'. I just couldn't get past those first few dates that would result in me finding my soulmate, that one person who could really help me on those rubbish days (and recycling days – why are there so many different coloured bins?). At one point, I thought I'd got close, but when things progressed to a more 'physical' connection I discovered he had back hair to rival Sasquatch, and as lovely as it might have been to combine spooning with practising my French-braiding skills, personally it just wasn't my bag. Surprising, considering my beast fetish. I wanted to find that missing person who completed me, not the missing link. Turns out, those years of unrealistic expectations had manifested into some pretty high self-sabotaging standards and a complete reluctancy to negotiate on some of the less important aspects standing in the way of a potential partnership. I believe the psychological term is 'a fussy bitch'.

Just when I was beginning to feel as though there was something wrong with EVERY SINGLE ONE of them, boom! Enter stage left, Mr Right. Tall, dark, chiselled, handsome, and with eyes as blue as my recycling bin. I shit you not, like Superman crossed with a Disney prince. Oddly enough, our first encounter was not on a speeding form of public transport, mid fighting the forces of evil, or on a Beverly Hills street corner in a cracking pair of fuck-me boots. No, it was how all the best, and non-Hollywood, love stories start of course: in a questionable night club, our love heightened by the aphrodisiacal and aromatic notes of alcopops and sick. As the cigarette smoke parted and Chesney Hawkes blared out at full blast, our eyes met. Him in jeans and a shirt, two pots of VO5 gel having made the ultimate sacrifice to fix his jet-black hair into position. Me in a black boob tube, teamed with a denim miniskirt and approximately 8,000 belts. Unable to move due to his magnetism and the weight of my accessories, I felt like we were the only two people in the room. He made his approach, and I tried to play it super cool, hoping the stench from my sweaty, streaky, fake tan wouldn't put him off. He was Steve, a physiotherapy student who'd clocked my broken wrist from a misjudged Malia foam party two weeks prior and used it as a perfect in to start the chat-up proceedings.

'Ulna?' he smouldered.

'Err, no, Sophie,' I sheepishly replied.

'No, your wrist. Have you broken your ulna?'

'Oh … no, scaphoid,' I cringed, awkwardly. WHAT. A. FUCKING. IDIOT. He belly laughed while I beamed a deep shade of crimson. Turned out, not only was he FIT, but he was kind, interesting, and didn't mention my tits once. It felt different – being in his presence made my heart race, my palms clammy, and my stomach somersault, although admittedly all also symptoms of too many sambuca shots. Was it love at first sight? I'm not entirely sure … but it was definitely lust, and not disgust, so I'd take it. For us star-crossed lovers, time stood still … and as Chesney blurred into Darude, and Darude into Guns N' Roses' 'Sweet Child o' Mine', I had already decided that if I was ever going to procreate, he might possibly be the sweet father of mine. Yes, I was 52 per cent certain he was 'the one', and in that moment I was just a girl, standing in front of a badly-dressed beaver … asking him for another Apple VK. Fucking magical.

Roll credits.

3

Matrimoany

Love and marriage go together like a ... horribly imposed societal expectation. It seems as though the minute you're in a relationship that lasts longer than a menstrual cycle, there's an idea you must pin your newly acquired partner down in a very difficult to wriggle out of, WWE-style, wed-lock. There are many who are all for going hard on the early doors commitment, and there are others, mainly Catherine Howard and Anne Boleyn, who'd retrospectively argue against making hasty decisions, instead opting to truly get to know a person's character and flaws before losing your head. Is your person someone you can love, and live with, forever? Getting married is a massive expense, and a huge pain in the arse. Nowadays, in a much more liberal world than good old Henry VIII's days, is it even relevant any more? Aside from a nice dress, six identical toasters, and fancy table centrepieces, what does a wedding bring to a couple? Because if that's all you're after, you can get the same joy in John Lewis but with the added benefit of a no-quibble return policy. You don't need to be married to live with someone, make babies, or have a giant piss-up with your mates. So, just posing the question here ... why do many of us still take the plunge?

Eighteen months after fate waved its mysterious and magical wand over a sticky-floored nightspot in Leeds, Steve and I were very much the poster children for smug, cohabiting 'happily ever after' twats. We'd packed up our northern love affair and moved down south to London to live out our highly ambitious career goals of making other people coffee for the minimum wage. Having begged, borrowed and stolen enough cash to buy our very first home together, we managed to nab a lovely little shoebox in a leafy garden city. We didn't have a garden ... but we were assured by people with more money than us that they were definitely there. Life was good! We were settled, enjoying our twenties in (OK, near ...) the hustle and bustle of the Big Smoke – so imagine my surprise when he decided to rock the boat with a VERY important question ...

'Are you sure?' I suspiciously questioned, jerking his face towards mine with both hands, scrupulously inspecting his face for telltale signs of piss-taking, uncertainty, or alcohol consumption.

'Of course I am! Are you?' He laughed, beaming at me.

'An all-inclusive trip to Thailand ... and you're paying? HELL TO THE YES!'

Truth be told, I hadn't even thought about a marriage proposal – not until I broke the news of our exotic and highly romantic vacation to my girlfriends over Soho cocktails that my office-bitch salary couldn't afford (there's a moral in the story about leaving university with a 2:2 in Pubic Relations).

'Oh my God, he's totally going to propose!' My friend Lorna squealed with excitement, already mentally planning the hen party and calibrating how many penis straws would be required.

No, he was not going to propose … was he? WAS HE?! He was, he totally was! It was the only logical explanation as to why two people, in a serious relationship, in rainy England would ever get on an aeroplane and go on holiday to a much warmer country. It was in this moment I realised … I actually wanted him to. But I was too young for marriage, right? Twenty-three. The idea was ludicrous; do non-seventeenth-century people, especially those not in the 'family way' do that? What about everything my 18-year-old self had said? But then, she was a big fan of hair mascara and body glitter, so potentially not the most trustworthy in terms of sound life advice. Yes, the more I thought about it, the less ridiculous the concept seemed in my head … I wasn't planning on dishing out any more oats, and I was perfectly happy with the one reliable turtle neck for the rest of my life. Maybe we *should* get married … WAIT. WHAT? How was I at that needy, 'contemplating the logistics of a crate of doves' point already? It really hadn't taken very long for me to succumb to the allure of tradition, security, and half his earnings. Maybe I should stand firmer for longer? Be more independent and embed some grounded feminist anti-patriarchy views into the situation? OR, I could be a real-life Disney princess on MY special day! And no, I'm not even going to correct myself there and say 'our' – he would be there to hold the rings and prop me up after too much cheap cava, like a bridegroom Billy bookcase. I did still wonder, though … how much of a difference a piece of paper would make to our relationship? Surely it wouldn't make me love him any more? I don't know, maybe it would … One thing was for sure: knowing it wouldn't be *as* easy for him to escape in the dead of night was certainly an appealing prospect.

So off we jetted, thirteen stopovers in countries I'd never heard of, until finally we arrived – wizened by economy time-travel, in beautiful … rainy Thailand. Monsoon season – apparently a great time of year to secure a cheap deal … but would it be the perfect opportunity to secure a lifetime contract?

I lived my life on the wet and slippery edge for the entirety of that holiday, constantly on high alert for proposals. In between torrential downpours, it was the ideal engagement location – white beaches, palm trees, passion as hot as the food. Every time he said my name I was expecting it to be followed up with '… will you marry me?' Instead, it was '… can you pass me another toilet roll?' Or, '… did you pack the Dioralyte?' Honestly, every time he bent double with a stomach cramp I thought my luck was in – poor lad, he was just trying not to shit himself. Romantic – albeit clenched – strolls on the beach were blighted by bitter disappointment – me fluttering my lashes at him, expectantly, him questioning whether I was having a seizure. It would have been my dream moment, apart from the fact it wasn't. Zip. Nada. Nothing. The only ring action was that of a man who'd consumed a questionable eight-hour-old Pad Thai from the all-you-can-eat buffet. It was only ten days later, during the six-hour layover in Kuwait airport, that it finally dawned on me … it probably wasn't going to happen, and that was fine. Wasn't it? No of course it wasn't, because as well as me feeling disappointed, I knew I'd be going home with disheartening news for other people too … mainly the dove man, and Lorna, who'd put in a girthy order for penis straws from China. Strapping my sensible head back on, I reasoned that in all honesty it was probably too soon – there were some mental images and smells that needed time to dissipate first. When our next trip came around five months later, a pre-Christmas jaunt to New York, my expectation level was zero and so I went armed with a guarded heart, and a handbag full of Imodium. This time, neither of us were going to be caught short.

Now, here's the thing about proposals – there's a lot of expectation put on the poor soul doing the asking, especially in the social media era. People live for the story, don't they? It's the first thing they ask after inspecting your finger to make sure the ring isn't as big as their own, or the one they gave their partner. 'How did he do it?' 'Did he get down on one knee?' 'Give us all the gory details!' The drama, the pressure, the oneupmanship of it all …

Something I was not aware of ahead of our trip stateside was that Steve was actually a better liar than I gave him credit for, because unbeknown to me he was indeed planning to propose. Now, let me tell you how I fucked it up …

Credit where credit is due, on a day when Bitchy McBitchface had gone nuclear at him for not putting together a chest of drawers he'd had a whole 10 hours to build while I was at work, he had actually driven all the way up to Liverpool to ask my dad's permission. Very old school that, isn't it? And something I'm still confused about – what's the need? Most women, especially, have been flipping their dads the proverbial 'V's since the age of 11. 'Can I go to town with my mates? No? Right, well I'm off through my bedroom window, so I'll see you at 3 a.m. in a pool of WKD Blue vomit.' Very suspiciously, my dad, big John, had agreed – presumably seeing an opportunity to rid himself of the financial burden of still having to slip me a twenty-pound note every time I visited.

Off we jetted to America, me blithely unaware of any of this, him shiftily passing through airport security with a face that said 'I've got 5 kg of cocaine stashed up my arse'. Turns out there was indeed some ring smuggling going on … but of the diamond variety.

After 48 hours sightseeing, shopping, and taking a million pictures of yellow taxis, he sprung it on me that we were going out to a super-fancy restaurant in the Meatpacking District. So, of course, I did as any self-respecting girl would do and embarked on a mission to see how many cosmopolitans I could down before needing a charcoal nightcap. Turns out, not that many. By the time we got to the restaurant, I no longer had the ability to see, so did not notice his incredibly anxious face, nor the super-attentive fancy waiter lurking by the table, ready to drop a diamond ring in my glass of bubbly. Nor was I aware of how loudly I was shouting across the table, 'BABE! BABE! ASK THEM FOR MORE BREAD!', or that I had completely lost the capacity to hear him respond that I'd already eaten the equivalent of twelve French sticks. After he had to assist/drag me to the ladies' room for a tactical vomit, the moment was well and truly gone, and by the end of the night, the only thing that was engaged was the toilet cubicle.

As a testament to his feelings towards me, he was not perturbed by my previous night's actions and was still very much determined to pop the big question in the Big Apple. If the shoe had been on the other foot, I would have been so furious I might have ended it there and then. Fortunately, he's a better person than I am, because the morning after, on our last day, he bought me beige salty carbs and suggested going for a romantic winter's stroll around a snow-covered Central Park. It was so beautiful, like a scene out of a Hollywood movie I'd always imagined myself in – except in this straight-to-DVD version I had to stop every couple of hundred metres to retch into a bin. Magical. As we paused at the famous Gapstow Bridge, I was so busy concentrating on breathing in deeply through my nose and out through my mouth that I hadn't clocked him on the ground – potentially mugged and stabbed, for all the attention I was paying. As I garbled on about a scene from *Home Alone 2* in a bid to convince us both that I was TOTALLY fine, I heard five completely unexpected words …

'Sophie … Will you marry me?'

The shock was so great that I could have thrown up, but fortunately there wasn't anything left in my stomach, so instead I regurgitated the most sentiment-filled response my dehydrated brain could muster …

'Shut up!'

Yes, I'd just told the penis of my dreams, who was currently on one knee, exposing his ring for all to see, to shut up. I then continued to tell him to shut up a further thirteen times (not that he counted and held it against me for years) before realising I hadn't actually given him an answer … which was of course, yes! If he was happy take me on in my current state then I really had bagged myself an absolute keeper.

So we were engaged! Time to plan a wedding – what fun! SAID NO ENGAGED PERSON EVER. Wedding planning, without a shadow of a doubt, is one of the most stressful experiences two human beings can put themselves through. On average, divorce happens eight years after the exchanging of vows – to be honest, I'm bloody amazed people actually make it as far as the aisle without blocking each other on Instagram and moving to opposite sides of the planet. I've got a suggestion for the FBI, CIA, MI6, etc. – if you really want to psychologically torture a terrorist into giving you information, just pass them a seating plan for 150 people who don't like each other, and a list of their dietary requirements. They'll sing like fucking canaries. Honestly, the number of conversations we had with various family members that went like this …

'Auntie Pam's a vegan, but she prefers not to eat mushrooms, so is there anything else on the menu she can have?'

'Yes … water.'

Why is it people think they can treat other people's weddings like a fancy restaurant, putting in their special food orders as though they're cruising through the McDonald's Drive-Thru. I'll give you some options, OK?

a) You get what you're given, and don't complain about it
b) You bring a cereal bar in your pocket, and you don't complain about it
c) You don't come, and you don't complain about it

In the end, we were effectively railroaded into a wedding banquet of chicken and two veg by the 'can't chew beef with my false teeth' cartel.

'Clive has asked whether he'll be able to bring his new lady friend, that he met in his local Tesco last week, as a plus one. Do you think that would be OK?'

'Sorry, Mum – who the fuck is Clive?'

Honestly, the amount of people who were snuck onto my wedding list like it was a secret VIP Justin Bieber gig was unreal. It gets SO political. With most people bound by venue capacity and budgets, if your name's not on the list, you ain't getting in. So who do you crop, without making parents from both sides of the family cry, and write you out of their wills? Well, firstly, the obvious choice is to get rid of the shouty ones who are bound to kick off during the speeches – no, not the groomsmen, the kids. Yes, the highly controversial no-children rule has been dividing wedding planning and causing friendship feuds since the dawn of time. People get VERY offended when you ban their offspring from YOUR big day – something I always found to be confusing, because normally parents are always banging on about how they can't wait to get rid of their kids for a few hours. Get a babysitter, get shitfaced, and be safe in the knowledge that the only bodily fluids you'll be cleaning up will be your own.

Next on the cull list … friends' partners who you've never met. Then there's the 'problem guests', the ones you really don't want to invite but you have been emotionally blackmailed into it by certain influential members of the family/firm.

'Your Dad's friend Nigel called and promised he absolutely won't do any class A drugs within forty-eight hours of the wedding, so can he come?' Yes, *those* family members who really should be in prison but somehow, up until that point, have managed to elude the system. They're only allowed to come on the proviso that they are supervised by your Nan at all times, and stand at the edge of all professional photography so they can be cropped out according to the severity of their inevitable criminal conviction.

You also have to consider the ones who you love dearly, but are going to have 10 drinks and go on an inebriated rampage of destruction. There's just something about the dangerous combination of a free bar, not being fed until the late afternoon, and then having to sit through hours of speeches (another discussion point), that lends itself so incredibly well to getting absolutely hammered and potentially ruining someone's big day. For example, my friend Jess – a perfectly rational and lovely person when sober – was so plastered at her brother's wedding, that for some reason, on all the professional pictures, she decided to grab hold of her hubby's penis as though it were a handheld detonator of an explosive device. Believe me when I say it was a bomb NO ONE wanted to go off. Put a completely different meaning behind the sentiment of 'to have and to hold'. Not only are you paying thousands of pounds for other people to embarrass themselves, but you're also paying through the nose to have people embarrass you. That's right, the speeches! Best men, ironically named, are there with the sole intention of stitching up the groom and making his new bride's mother weep with horror at stories of her son-in-law's past sexual conquests and questionably exotic masturbation habits. Ah, precious memories, awkward future family gatherings, and a heavily overdrawn bank account … but is it really worth it?

I was forever seeing bridal magazines with all these happy, beautiful and beaming brides-to-be and after a year of planning I could only assume it was because they were on whatever Nigel was smoking. There are just so many decisions to make, and if you, like me, are a person who finds decisiveness somewhat challenging, wedding planning can feel like a never-ending nightmare episode of *The Crystal Maze*. Honestly, the whole process had me questioning whether marriage was really all it was cracked up to be. Steve and I were averaging an argument every thirty-three seconds, I hadn't spoken to my mum in over four weeks over a disagreement surrounding a chair cover, and my dad had completely lost the plot over the importance of a well-balanced canapé platter. Instead of coming together over the bond of love and happiness, we were all unravelling at the seams of very expensive formal wear. Speaking of which, I found shopping for my gown incredibly stressful – turns out finding 'the dress' is just as difficult as finding 'the one'. I honestly thought I'd put one on, a chorus of angels would appear and my friends would sob at my breathtaking beauty and radiance. No, none of that. By the 756th dress I tried on, I was ready to get married in one of my mum's fitted sheets, with a crocheted blanket veil like I'd practised as a kid. Eventually, and heavily influenced by Ariel, I settled on a lace mermaid tail, which was nice but never felt 'destined'. It also proved I'd learnt absolutely nothing from the age of six, because how the hell was I going to go for a poo?

Another highly political part of the whole process is the ceremonial selection and inauguration of the bridal bodyguards, the penis-straw posse, the wedding party high priestesses – otherwise known as the bridesmaids. It's their big moment, their time to shine and strut down that aisle like pastel-chiffon-clad Pussycat Dolls. But how do you go about picking the band members from your trusted and much-loved girl gang? AND, which one do you choose to be leader of the pack? You're always going to offend someone, aren't you? It's contentious. You could just ask some cute young kids to be your flower girls instead, apart from ... oh wait ... you banned them all from your wedding. However difficult it might be, it can be navigated effectively by getting really drunk and asking whichever of your friends is standing closest to you at the time. 'I bloody luv you!'

Once chosen, it's not all plain sailing for the bridesmaids; yes, they get their moment of glory on the big day but it comes at great sacrifice – planning the hen party. Best bit about being a bride is that you can have absolutely no part in that fuck-awful logistical nightmare (if you have any common sense) – make your pissed selection then just walk away and let them deal with the 7,000 emails from overly excited and opinionated women. One thing's for sure, you'll always end up in a dance studio above a kebab shop learning the routine to 'Single Ladies'. It's not what you'd have chosen, but it matters not, because it's not about you – you just have to run with it and go all in. You're either SWAT (Sloshed Women Away Together), or you're not. I decided to have my pre-marital send-off the same weekend that Steve was on his stag – no bloody way I was sitting at home twiddling my thumbs while he and thirty of his KNOBS (not an acronym) headed off on a three-day bender to Eastern Europe. No, I would be living my best life learning a Beyoncé dance, while he lived his ... getting a lap dance. Fuck's sake. I dread to think what actually happens on stag parties. Partners definitely get the PG-13 highly edited version of events on their return. Do we even want to know? My friend's soon-to-be husband actually ended up confessing everything after the 'no touching' rule in a strip club landed him in VERY hot water. Poor lad tried to go 'contactless' but an entrepreneurial exotic dancer had other plans ... using his Apple Pay to swindle him out of £600. He then had to go home and tell his fiancée he'd 'stripped' the joint account of their wedding funds paying another woman to shake her boobs in his face. Even worse, he got kicked out before getting the dance. Bad times. It's not just men who get themselves into trouble, though; us women have a knack of being just as badly behaved as our male counterparts ... the differential point is we're just not stupid enough to get caught. Although there were no incidents of credit-card fraud, my hen was full of misdemeanours, more penis straws than you could shake a dick at, fabulous girliness, a near-drowning incident, the drunken hijacking of yacht, the loss of several toenails, a LOT of laughs and, of course ... oh, oh, oh, oh-oh, oh ... *THAT* sodding dance.

Once the hen and stag parties are out of the way, and everyone has returned with all their limbs and eyebrows intact, it's downhill to the big day! Cakes, corkage, DJs ... Have you picked your dance-floor playlist? What about the first dance? Steve and I had no romantic attachments to any particular song, and to say our tastes in music differed somewhat was an understatement – we had a two-hour argument over whether or not Eminem's 'Stan' should really be a part of our special day. I loved him dearly, but up until that point his contribution had been picking the honeymoon (potentially a bargain deal to the Caribbean, in hurricane season), so to come at me with a shouty dude in a white vest talking about a murdering superfan was like a red rag to an already high-maintenance bridezilla. 'STEVE – HOW'S MY NAN SUPPOSED TO DANCE TO SLIM?!'

I think there's also a fear, when you get so close, that things might just go horribly wrong all in the final throes. I was convinced he was going to do a runner, or leave me jilted at the altar. I made him promise that, whatever happened, he'd go through with the day so that I could save face, and that we could just get it annulled afterwards – secretly knowing he'd never get round to doing the paperwork.

The night before the big day, I was back at my parents' house, a complete nervous wreck, and sharing a bed with my big sister – who'd also brought her cat back with her for the occasion, as you do. I know people listen to rain music, whale sounds, crashing waves on a beach to get to sleep, but I can categorically state that listening to a tabby cat take a shit in a pile of scented gravel is not on that list for a very good reason. The morning consisted of prepping, preening, realising going for a double-dip spray tan was a bad idea, massively stressing about EVERYTHING, and drawing straws with my bridesmaids as to who was going to help me go to the toilet while wearing my lacy intestine-compressing outfit. This of course was all going on as a wedding photographer casually perched on the end of my bed with a telescopic lens saying, 'Just pretend I'm not here!' It would have been easier to ignore herpes.

Why is the morning of your wedding so absolutely bowel-liquidisingly terrifying? In theory, it's meant to be right up there as one of the happiest days of your life … you're no longer on that dusty shelf batting off social commentary about not getting any younger. It should be very jolly and lovely – you're marrying the love of your life. So why the feeling of dread, nervousness, and nausea? I was absolutely bricking it. What if he wasn't there? What if one of the groomsmen had shaved off his hair the night before? My biggest fear was an Eastern European stripper coming down the aisle with a baby bump and card-reading machine doing her best Marshal Mathers. 'Hey, Steve, I wrote … but you're still not calling!'

Fortunately, for all our sakes, he was there, and as our vows nervously tumbled out of our mouths, the stress and the strains of the past eighteen months melted away. The arguments, the politics, the seat covers and canapés paled into insignificance …

It was just the two of us, promising to have and to hold each other, for better or worse, in sickness … and in hangovers, to love and to cherish, until death – or a fight about whose parents we'd spend Christmas with– us do part. And do you know what? In that moment – I didn't even think it was possible – the love I had for my new husband grew. I don't know where it snuck in from, like a romance ninja, because I certainly wasn't expecting it – but yes, out of nowhere we found another sneaky 10 per cent we didn't know we had. There are those – matrimony cynics and miseries – who say marriage is just a piece of paper, what difference can it make to a relationship? For us however, I feel as though it cemented our bond and took us to another level.

Unfortunately, it also took my friend Jess to another place too, this time not to her husband's trouser grenade but to A&E after tripping over my Nan's walking stick while dancing to 'Stan'. I managed to emotionally hold myself together throughout the day too, until the moment we said goodbye to our guests and headed up to our suite to 'make things official', which unfortunately coincided nicely with the onset of my post-wedding blues. Highly triggered by the taking off of my dress and realising never again would I be a sexy Disneyesque siren bride, I cried for three weeks straight, leaving Steve to question whether he'd made the right decision by being 'part of my world'.

OK, so where am I at here? Having come out the other side of the actual process of holy matrimoany – is it all it's cracked up to be? Is it worth the anxiety, arguments, and anticlimax? THE BLOODY MONEY? Personally, and of course it's a very personal choice, I'm going out on a limb and saying, to me, yes it was. I enjoyed getting married (eventually) – standing there in front of our family and friends, publicly making those lifelong vows, cemented what we had. It made us feel unbreakable, unstoppable, and unified. Ask anyone, though, and they'll say marriage is more than a wedding, more than one day in a nice dress and making a scary commitment out loud. It's bloody hard work, it requires compromise, and taking the time to show one another – day in, day out – that you meant what you said standing there at that altar. It's messy, it's mundane, you may neglect one another, and the passion may very well run dry. Sometimes it works, sometimes it doesn't – sometimes you lose yourself, sometimes you're found. The important thing to remember is that it's a journey of sharing … your heart, soul, worries, and student debts. Thanks for that, Steve. Halfsies on the £9k I pissed up the wall on shoes and booze is MASSIVELY appreciated!

4

Grumpy-Pumpy

Eggs are not my forte – scrambled, soft boiled, poached, and arguably the most terrifyingly challenging of them all … fertilised.

There comes a time in adulthood when you arrive at a life-altering crossroad. To baby, or not to baby? That is the question. This junction can either propel you towards a dazzling moment of clarity, or it can devour you whole, spitting you out into an existential crisis that leaves you highly conflicted as to how ready you are to give up your freedom, binge-drinking, and lie-ins. Which way do you turn though? Down a safe and familiar trodden path, or, do you take a leap of faith and plummet headfirst into the unknown and shit-scary world of parenthood?

When our first baby arrived, I wasn't prepared in the slightest for the colossal upheaval to our formerly carefree lifestyle. The constant crying, sleepless nights, incessant demand for food, toilet-training … or lack of. Yes, Millie, our ten-week-old beagle puppy, well and truly made her mark on our lives … sofa, carpet, and king-sized mattress. We were walking clichés, guilty of doing what so many couples unsure of their parenting abilities had done before us, and had decided to first try our hand at caring for the canine species before being let loose on our own. But she wasn't just any dog … no, no. She was a bloody-tampon-stealing, poo-rolling-in, Houdini-esque havoc hound whose sole purpose in life was to pillage bins as though she was Indiana Jones in *Raiders of the Lost Bark*. Edible or not, she'd give it a good crack. It was very similar to living with The Very Hungry Caterpillar – if it'd hatched with two fewer legs, sprouted fur, and had the ability to clear rooms with a fart. On Monday she ate an apple … device (an iPad to be precise); on Tuesday she ate two pairs … of shoes; on Wednesday she ate three plum-coloured cushions; on Thursday she ate four straw laundry baskets; on Friday she ate five chocolate oranges; and on Saturday headed straight to the out-of-hours vet, at a cost of £1,500.

As much trouble as she was, she was my baby and I loved that fluffy hell-raiser as only a deluded mother could. 'She's not naughty, Steve, she's a free spirit!' When we went to pick her, she was the only one in the litter who was awake, quietly sitting on her own in the corner of the pen. She trotted over to us with her big brown eyes full of love, cute black tail, complete with white tip, wagging in delight, and she totally had me. Opting for a beagle over most other breeds because of their eternal cuteness, I'd massively overlooked the vast majority of their dominant traits, such as stubbornness, greed, and horrific wind. It took me three months to realise she was effectively me, in dog form. Our first attempts at discipline and asserting our parental dominance were met with the middle claw, and so we quickly outsourced to puppy training school – an awkward six weeks of watching other people's dogs do as they were told while she ran around hump-ing and stealing things. I'm pretty certain they only let us pass in order to get rid of us – as a testament to this, we have an amazing picture of her eating the graduation rosette as her final 'fuck you' to the establishment. If anything, instead of preparing me for motherhood, she actually just uncovered all of my potential parenting flaws and highlighted how much of a bad mother I'd be. Regularly allowing her to prey on my weaknesses – a sucker for sad eyes, and totally obsessed with the need for her to love me – I was a complete pushover. That said, in terms of a controlled experiment, puppy ownership semi-served its purpose: we loved her, played with her, remembered to feed and water her, and – unlike our failed houseplant venture – managed to keep her alive (despite her best efforts to digest non-edible materials).

SURELY looking after a baby would be easier than a puppy? Presumably a child would be at least *one* before it could eat its way through the Christmas tree lights, consume its own faeces, or shred a duck faster than a waiter at a Chinese restaurant. Yes, I now knew *exactly* the type of mother I was going to be to a human baby – shouty, gagging at sloppy poo, emotionally needy, and with zero qualms about rewarding bad behaviour with snacks.

Now, as a newlywed, there are two certainties in life. The first is that you'll discover a devastating fact about your new spouse after it's too late to do anything about it (Steve, for example, has a horrifyingly differing Father Christmas belief system to my own – he grew up thinking parents send gifts to Santa, in advance, which he then delivers back to children on their behalf … WHAT?! It makes no sense man! What about the elves in the workshop? The carbon footprint of it? MADNESS!) The second is that people will feel the need to ask you very openly about when you plan to start having unprotected sex and use your bodily fluids to make humans. Sorry, *what now*? How very weird, very intrusive, and none of your bloody business. I often wonder whether the problem lies in an inability to form interesting conversation once the weather has already been discussed, or that they're just blighted by insensitivity and ignorance. Folks have a tendency to wade on in there with their size elevens, completely disregarding those who don't feel ready, who are trying, who can't, or those who have lost ... and what about those who simply don't want them and shouldn't have to explain themselves to every Tom, Dick and Harry who wants to know the literal 'ins and outs' of their foofs.

Motherhood is a scary prospect that's not for everyone. It isn't a defining characteristic of womanhood, it's a chapter – one some choose to dive head first into, while others are more than happy to skip it altogether, opting to read ahead to the next part of their story, totally empowered by their own choices and narrative. I was in neither of these camps, sitting somewhere between intrigued and horrified. The whole prospect of actually going 'yes let's do this!' felt completely alien (I was also worried that's what would come out of me). In a way, trying for children felt almost like an inevitability ... a fate unlikely to be dodged. I loved Steve, and the idea of seeing little versions of ourselves running around, albeit terrifying and a tad narcissistic, was realistically the next exciting step in our relationship. A year after tying the knot, we'd quit our jobs and travelled the world for a year – we'd lived our best lives and so it was probably the right time to just crack on with the act of making some. When we finally decided to take the plunge into parenting, despite our practice run with the dog, I still wasn't actually fully ready. I mean, who really is? Especially if it's your first, it's the complete unknown, and it's SCARY. Also, there's no such a thing as 'the right time' when it comes to finding space in your life for children. It's totally different for blokes – they don't have to grow them and birth them ... it's one small(er) step for man, and one giant-headed baby coming out of our vaginas for womankind.

What if there was something wrong with my (OK, our …) baby? What if I grew the antichrist? What if I didn't love it? And it didn't love me, growing up and attempting to divorce me like Macaulay Culkin did to his parents? What if it was NOT a cute baby but I was one of *those* mothers who couldn't see it and proudly sent pictures of a double-chinned potato, complete with a pink bow glued to its head, to my local newspaper's 'Bonny Baby' competition? If I had a boy, I would be growing a penis inside me. A PENIS! I wasn't sure how I felt about that either. And do not get me started on the notion of a real-life thing living inside me, taking up squatters' rights then trying to smash its way through my front (bottom) door à la Jack Nicholson in *The Shining*. *'Should have used a Johnny!'*

Managing to put my fears of Beelzebubba to one side, we decided it was time to give it a go. I could have talked myself out of it a million times over, but I had to look at the bigger life-picture … if we didn't procreate, when I was 85 who was going to do my Tesco big shop for me?

As it happens, we ended up having two babies – and as yet, the world has not collapsed into a cavernous, fiery hell pit patrolled by demonic footmen. The journey of how those two bundles of joy – Jack (I GREW A PENIS!) and Evelyn – came to enter the world, however, was not quite as easy as I'd anticipated. You see, it turns out baby making was not as easy as I had been led to believe. Sod's Law says if you're a carefree teenager throwing contraception caution to the wind, then you're likely to be a fertile goddess. As an adult woman, besieged by the stresses of the modern world, with a habit of overanalysing everything, and a hefty caffeine addiction, then it can sometimes be a slightly different story.

Who knew making humans was so complex? It's genuinely mind-boggling we even exist as a species and that the first humans thousands of years ago didn't just give up, go fucking nuts in a Pleistocene Ibiza and, then die out. There's a completely new language to decipher, and after a quick search of a few baby forums, I was more confused than when watching *Line of Duty*. Seriously, there were so many words and acronyms I'd legitimately NEVER heard of. 'Basal', for example, I presumed was somewhere in Switzerland – not, in fact, a way of recording your body temperature to track fertility. 'Follicular' I wrongly presumed was a reason why men use caffeine shampoo, but no! Apparently it's the time between the first day of your period and ovulation. 'SMEP' – not a fancy brand of fridge but, according to my newly acquired GCSE (Google-Created Sexual Education), a 'sperm meets egg plan'. 'DPO' was another one … 'day past ovulation' in case you didn't know – not to be confused with a delivery service (although if I could have got a baby sent to me next-day, that would have made life easier). I was a complete conception virgin (CCV).

If it was this difficult to make them, how hard would it be to raise them?! You spend so much of your young adult life trying not to get pregnant, there's an assumption the minute you remove contraception your womb will succumb faster than your dieting willpower when faced with a bag of salty and delicious Kettle Chips, but this is not always the case. I look back at my early twenties' belt-and-braces approach of using the pill, a condom, and a picture of a potato baby on my bedside table, and it's laughable. In reality, it's easier to make a baked Alaska than it is to make a baby. HOT ICE CREAM, people. Let that sink in.

The pressing point here is the 'con' that is conception. We're all fed this ideology that the process of reproduction is a beautiful experience, sprinkled with a dash of Harry Potter wizardry. Well, let me tell you this … there wasn't much magic in the house of Hufflemuff – just ovulation kits, and a tick list of Google's best insemination tactics. Yes, when it comes to trying for a baby, there's a definite 'misconception' of the 'fun' element, unless you happen to get your kicks out of charting cervical mucus – a hobby which, sadly, comes with several strings attached. Steve thought it'd be months of top-notch randy shagging – not me eerily floating out of the bathroom in my hooded bathrobe, a horrible sense of misery and foreboding in the room as I leant in to give him my Dementor's kiss ... seductively whispering in his ear, 'I've got my egg whites'. Poor lad now has an eye twitch at the mere mention of a pavlova, and don't EVER ask him if he wants an Eton mess.

Yes, unsexy sex! The downfall of most couples embarking on the Great British Bonk Off. The idea of relentless shagging is super appealing at first, but several months into the process, rumpy-pumpy all too soon turns into grumpy-pumpy – especially when the very height of romance is considered merely acknowledging one another before stripping off only the bare essentials in order to get the job done. Socks and top-half items must always remain on in order to complete this soul-destroying part of the proceedings. What was once an amorous, intimate expression of love between partners can become a process, a chore, as formulaic as algebra – and that takes its toll on even the healthiest of relationships. Post-coital cuddles are replaced with bat-like practices of hanging from the bed frame by your ankles, spontaneity exchanged for precisely planned positions, *'No babe, pivot ... PIVOT!'* Not to mention the added pressure of functional fornication – performing for an actual reason – and after so many years of practising in the 'undressed' rehearsal, showtime can often lead to sexy-time stage fright for both parties. You also have to contend with everyone else being an expert on the matter of how best your other half should impregnate you ...

'Missionary is best, allows for all those strong swimmers to really get right on in there!' Thanks for that, now knob off, Nan.

'OK dear, but what about doggie?'

'We leave her outside ...'

I had no idea that there was such a small window in which you can actually get pregnant; it's about six days a month – and even then it's not overly likely fertilisation will occur in the given time frame. Where was this information in high school? In retrospect, my Church of England girls' school probably didn't want us all knowing how statistically small the chances of pregnancy were – otherwise the Year 11 disco with the local boys' school would have been absolute carnage. I can just imagine our stern headmistress's stance on the matter. 'Look at Mary, girls, she was a virgin and she still got caught out. Keep your wits, and tits, about you!' Mary was bloody lucky that the first coming involved no coming, and that she relied on divine intervention instead of uterine.

For us non-chosen ones, a life of piss sticks, shovelling down multi-vitamins and pureed pond-slime smoothies awaits. It's not just us gals who suffer either … during our periods of trying, Steve's coffee was removed, alcohol consumption scrutinised, briefs replaced by boxers, and standing by the microwave was strictly forbidden.

After all the effort you've put into optimising hook-up conditions for your gametes, the two-week 'am I, aren't I?' limbo before seeing whether or not they've swiped left for each other can seriously mess with your mind. The obsessive googling of very early baby symptoms while desperately searching for proof of life can be all-consuming. *Horrific-smelling wind … am I pregnant? Incredibly annoyed by husband … am I pregnant? Ate three Big Macs and two family-sized bars of Dairy Milk … am I pregnant?*

So when a visit from your least favourite relative, Aunt Flo, arrives and pisses all over your phantom pregnancy parade it can be utterly devastating; firstly because you're not with child, and the hours of daytime acrobatics and burning urethra, have been in vain; secondly, the extra weight gain is all you (with a little help from the golden arches); and thirdly, you only have a week to mentally regroup before the whole emotional roller coaster happens all over again.

Every time I didn't 'pass' the highly anticipated pregnancy test, feelings of failure and inferiority bubbled to the surface – I'd see pregnant women out and about and feel a mixture of jealously, anger, and also intrigue … would it be socially acceptable to ask a total stranger how they did it? Was it a particular position, or technique … too forward? Or maybe backwards would be better … reverse cowgirl?! Did they have a secret code they could share with me, like a friend-referral voucher?

Now, here's the real Harry Potter magic: seeing the two red lines on that pee stick instead of the heart-wrenchingly disappointing singular one. Circumstances depending, it can be one of the most special, heart-hugging, romantic occasions a couple can share with one another … if you haven't happened to have just had a massive fight in a foreign country that's left you so enraged your piss is boiling (for once, not from cystitis). Yes, our first special 'magic moment' occurred on what had been a rather lovely holiday to Portugal's sunny Algarve, up until I opened the hire-car door into a lamp post that literally came from nowhere, causing more friction than an un-lubed hand job. It was only while sitting at a bar in a picturesque cobbled town – facing opposite directions, and pretending we didn't know one another – that it dawned on me I was probably so angry because I was premenstrual. After five confused minutes of counting and recounting on my fingers, I realised my period was AWOL by about a week. *No. Way.* Now, we all have flaws in our personalities, and one of mine is never wanting to break the ice after an argument – I'm happy to let the silence run for an eternity (or until he apologises for something that's my fault). On this occasion, due to extenuating circumstances, I was going to have to be the one who begrudgingly initiated the UN (Ultra Nervous) peace talks. So off we went in search of a test, things still frosty enough we could have ice skated our way to the town's incredibly stern-faced 700-year-old pharmacist who looked quite judgemental as I stood there phonically sounding out the words 'PR-EGG-NAN-CEEEEEE T-E-SSSSSSS-T' and partaking in a horrible sexually orientated game of charades.

Armed with a test, and a somewhat lost in translation pack of antibiotics, we headed back to the hotel. I really wasn't expecting a positive … so much so that after weeing half on the stick and half on my hand, I casually tossed it on the bathroom shelf and returned to the bedroom to continue with my passive aggression. I didn't *feel* remotely pregnant, so in my highly scientific mind, I obviously wasn't – I'd probably just confused my dates, or miscounted on my unreliable abacus fingers. Five or so minutes passed, and I was mid tucking into an extortionately priced miniature tub of hotel Pringles when Steve reminded me I should probably go and check the results before planning my evening's pina colada schedule. Nonchalantly strolling into the bathroom, humming to myself about being caught in the rain, I picked it up to see … one line. Not pregnant. I came out of the bathroom, threw the test at Steve and steadied myself for another month of the slightly less tropical non-stop penis collider. He looked down at the test, a look of confusion spreading across his face, and said, 'But what's this line?'

'It means no baby …' I replied, with an exasperated tut.

'I realise that one does … but what about the faint one next to it?'

'What do you mean faint one?' I squawked, rushing over to him to snatch my own urine-covered highlighter pen out of his hands. You had to squint to see it, but it was there … TWO. FECKING. LINES.

After hours of Google translating the test's Portuguese instruction leaflet, I lay in bed that night, trying to process the information I'd received only hours earlier. Pregnant. I kept running through it, over and over again in my mind. I was actually 'with' child, this is *exactly* how Mary must have felt after the Angel Gabriel delivered the good news. I also wondered whether Joseph had inconsiderately bought a bottle of champagne too, consuming it all before passing out and snoring loudly while she had a Fanta Lemon. I was only four weeks pregnant – by Dr Google's calculations, our baby was only the size of a poppy seed, but by some incredible feat of biological engineering had already developed all the building blocks required for growing into a real-life human being … It was absolutely mind-blowing, and freaky – very freaky. What was it doing in there? What were its motives? I'd had prawns for lunch, followed by a shot of port – had I damaged it? Even though this dot of a heroin seed was, in theory, a teeny tiny collection of cells, my fascination with it had well and truly begun. What would the future hold for him or her, and what about names? Regardless of what actually happened next with the pregnancy, a chain reaction had started, completely altering the course of my future, and my internet search history. It may have been yet to develop a heart, but like a pregnant Mr Grinch, mine, along with my tits, had already grown three times in size. I was all in.

At the time, the act of making a baby seemed like HARD graft, but retrospectively I was so lucky with my pregnancies, especially Jack's because he really didn't take as long as he could have done. His sister, being a typical girl, was trickier and arrived on the scene after what felt like a lifetime of constant trying, ovulation kits, and tears. With every month that passed I was left with a horrible sense of uneasiness … What if Jack had been a fluke? What if I'd used up all my good eggs? Why was conceiving second time round so much harder when we'd done everything the same as with our first? At times it was a dark and testing journey, one 18-year-old me never thought she'd venture on, but in the end our efforts were rewarded and I'll always appreciate how incredibly fortunate we are to have had that happy ending. It's amazing how the fertility journey differs from woman to woman, and how, give or take, we're all roughly made the same, though our experiences vary so much. I was definitely guilty of taking my eggs for granted, assuming my reproductive system would be ready and waiting, after years of being repressed by hormones, for the minute I decided to release my offspring into the world. Some are lucky enough to fall pregnant straight away; for others it takes months, even years; some are desperate to conceive and face cycle after cycle of IVF – heartache after heartache. There are those who'll never be able to carry a child of their own, while many, no matter the contraceptive barriers in place, discover that life just seems to find a way regardless. Planning, waiting, disappointment, arguments, heartbreak, and searching for ways to change vaginal pH balances – the desire to put all your love into another human being is as great as it is encompassing. Yes, motherhood may not be a defining characteristic of womanhood, or even adulthood, but for those who find themselves deeply immersed in its subtext it's a book that, once started, you can never truly put down.

The baby-making 'Game of Moans' can be difficult and totally unenjoyable, and do you know what? It's absolutely OK to admit that! It is FINE to say you hated trying to make a baby. You are not going to hell for that … in fact, your future children, when they come to understand how the birds and the bees work, will actually thank you for literally having no fun whatsoever when it came to creating their stroppy teenage lives. Pat yourself on the back, my friend, because you have already excelled in the first stages of parenting.

5

From Hump to Bump

Knocked up, preggers, up the duff, in the family way, a parasitic host ... however you want to describe it, life has changed BIG TIME. With a positive test result comes a whole mixed bag of feelings, something I refer to as the four 'H's of pregnancy: happiness, hesitancy, hysteria, and hunger. It was the highly anticipated moment I'd been waiting for most of my adult life – a valid reason to eat a whole tub of Ben & Jerry's at 2 a.m.

It's such a beautiful and special time. The joy you'll experience at demanding your partner constantly brings you carbs is unrivalled – 'BABY WANTS IT!' It may, however, be offset by some pretty serious post-conception concerns. There's been a major commitment to something you're not entirely sure you're going to like, similar to visiting the hairdresser's and asking for a fringe. You're worried about what people will think, feel sick to the stomach, and it's going to take months to grow. Yes, as exciting as the prospect of meeting your gorgeous gametes is, the pregnancy journey is long, tiring and often paved with panty liners.

Welcome to Panicsville, population: you. What about miscarriage, a problem with the baby, or me? What if I die, or, as initially feared, am carrying a murderous antichrist that'll eat its way out of the womb and then devour the world? That peed-on stick changes *everything* (hopefully for the best, apocalypse aside).

After determining when your due date is, and how far along you are, it's time to discover what joys the first trimester has in store. You may do as I did, after my first positive result, and book yourself in to see the doctor. Anyone else think it's majorly weird that medical professionals just take your word for it – no one actually checks, or asks for proof of your pregnancy until circa twelve weeks. Very trusting – I mean, you could be the village crazy and rock up at your scan with a cat shoved up your jumper. Apart from the test that claimed I was (but what if it was a false positive?!), one of my first pregnancy symptoms was burning areolas that'd seemingly been replaced with 'fresh from the grill' sized burger nips. For a lot of ladies, great-boob-balls-of-fire are one of the first indications of pregnancy. Walking up and down stairs, knocking our newly inflated knockers with a hairbrush, wearing a bra, not wearing a bra, sleeping on your front, sleeping on your side, sleeping on your back. You get the gist. My poor husband – it was the closest he'd ever got (in real life) to seeing porn-star boobs and if he'd dared lay a finger on them I'd have cut off his hands, frozen them, then used them as ice packs for my bra. Never mind fun bags, mine were closer to nun bags. Totally off limits.

Another of the big hitters for me was 'morning' sickness, which, by the way, needs an immediate rebrand to 'any time it fucking feels like it' sickness. Horrendous, and with Jack it started at thirteen weeks – relentlessly lasting all the way to twenty-seven weeks. Effectively, it was a lingering hangover but without any of the fun of going out, getting hammered, picking a fight with your front door, and then falling asleep on the floor spooning the dog. With Evelyn, it hit me pretty much at the same time as realising my period was late – the excessive saliva in my mouth was not only a key giveaway, but also prompted that age-old debate of 'spit or swallow?' Soon after drippy gob kicked in, my stomach contents kicked out – uncontrollably for months. One minute I'd be fine, the next I was vomiting all over myself while doing 70 mph down the M62. Weeks were spent with my head in toilets, bushes, gutters, buckets, or car foot-wells. One particularly awful time, it was so bad I couldn't drive myself to work, prompting Steve to very chivalrously take me in his car instead. As lovely as this gesture was, neither of us had had the foresight to move all the sick receptacles over from my vom vehicle to his, so ten minutes into the journey, when the need to chuck my guts up arose, there were zero waterproof options. Desperately searching for something girthier than my ankle boot, the only thing in sight was the box of Rice Krispies I'd brought along with me to serve as a bland all-day-breakfast buffet. Now, what would have made sense would have been to empty the cereal from the inner bag into the box then vomit into the impervious plastic. What I actually decided on, in the panic of the moment, was to remove the plastic bag completely and throw up into the highly permeable and extremely leaky cardboard box. Having not told anyone at work about the preggo situation, I could hardly walk into the office brandishing my soggy box of Snap, Crackle, and Puke, so I left it in Steve's capable hands to dispose of. Little did I know, he'd forget to do this and it would remain exactly where I'd left it when he collected me later. Funnily enough, the aroma of nine-hour-old sick didn't help my weak constitution. As it happens, revenge is a dish best served at 37.6°C, as once again his black sports car was transformed into the Batmo-bile. Quite possibly one of the worst experiences of my pregnancy career. This situation would have been completely avoidable, however, if only a ginger nut had been to hand … the least helpful morning sickness advice going, by the way. I've never snorted cocaine, but I imagine the burn is similar to that of having partially digested spicy complex carbohydrates stuck in your nasal passage. Anyone offering a biscuit during such a highly difficult digestive period deserves all the hormonal rage that's about to be projectile vomited in their general direction. There's a reason women in hospital with severe hyperemesis gravidarum aren't hooked up to an intravenous line of McVities … it just adds a festive, mulled-wine element to the sick.

With your first trimester comes a bit of a love–hate relationship with food. Is it a feeling of sickness, or hunger? It can become your arch nemesis if nothing will stay down, or a best friend if you're battling eternal hunger. My cravings were completely different in each pregnancy; with Jack, if it was salty and beige I was on it like a dog on chips. While carrying Evelyn, grapefruits, red peppers, and anything sour floated my boat along with – randomly – big juicy cucumbers … sadly for my husband, his was not included. Being pregnant, I discovered, is very similar to being a superhero: same amount of elasticated clothing, and the gift of actual real-life powers, such as being able to grow people, double in size, and detect a bag of crisps from fifty miles away. Working harder than a sniffer dog in an Australian airport, the pregnancy nose heightens *everything* – has the world always smelt so absolutely … godawful? For anyone struggling with what to buy a pregnant person for Christmas, a slogan T-shirt saying 'What's that funny smell?' should do nicely.

Combine all of the above with feeling totally overwhelmed, and a rampaging tidal wave of progesterone and oestrogen, and it's easy to see how expectant mothers can occasionally be an incy wincy bit on the emotionally tetchy side of life – especially when questioned on the validity of their feelings …

'STOP TELLING ME IT'S MY BASTARD HORMONES!' From narky to narcoleptic, everything seems so much more of an effort when your body is multiplying cells faster than an excel spreadsheet. You can hardly keep your eyes open; out for lunch, at the park with friends, or on a date night – boozing is replaced with snoozing. Now feels a good time to note the difference between your first pregnancy and your second … because first time round, if I felt knackered and wanted to lie down and rest, I just did. That was it, end of story. A lovely little nana nap for one. Second time round, the moment my head hit the pillow, I got tea-bagged by a kid in a shitty nappy who, if they could coherently speak, would say, 'Sleep when you're dead, bitch!'

When you're already a mum, there's no time to lie around, basking in the glory of being Queen Pregular the First and getting fussed over and hand-fed like a pregnant Labrador. There's work to be done – mounds of washing, endless food shops, nursery drops, tactical voms into bushes – all while a toddler hangs off your hip eating your hair. Also, no one really cares all that much … the glory days of being 'special' have well and truly gone. Remember when people held doors open for you, lifted all your heavy items, and it was absolutely acceptable to be a total bitch to anyone in your presence? 'Get me a bastard Snickers. NOW! Cheers, Gran.' Second baby, hello *Grease 2* of the sequel world! You're not the one anyone wants. You've already done it once, what are you expecting – a Pride of Britain award in the shape of a placenta? You're ravaged by tiredness, and there are no pregnancy compliments like the first-timers get, either. 'Oh, Susan's positively glowing!' Oh, fuck off, that's because Susan's had a twelve-hour sleep and a maternity massage. Meanwhile, the poor seasoned pros are just shuffling around as though we're sleep-deprived Ozzy Ozbournes, smacked off our tits on Vicks VapoRub and drenched in sweat from wrestling small human beings into car seats.

'Weeks' is a word you come to live by throughout this period, and even sometime after your child enters the world – until a friend has a much-needed word. 'Babe, he's not 418 weeks, he's eight years old. Let it go.' Weeks, you see, equate to milestones, and also very randomly to fresh produce that your growing embryo is meant to be equivalent to. Instagram is full of happy yet delirious-looking people lovingly holding mangos over their muffs. But regardless of how many babies you've had, the twelve-week mark is a particularly pivotal moment in your journey because for a lot of people it's the first opportunity to see for themselves that much-sought-after vital 'proof of life'. A wee-covered stick might say 'positive', and those lava lady lumps may be burning holes in your far-too-tight bra, but you're still not truly convinced your body is telling the truth. With both of mine, I was absolutely convinced they were phantom pregnancies, similar to what dogs have, and in another week I'd be carrying dolls round in my mouth and shredding newspaper under a table.

For me, the scan was my first chance for someone to confirm I wasn't suffering some kind of canine delusion. As well as the excitement at seeing your baby for the first time, you're also scared … will it be possible to get through the appointment without fetish-squirting two pints of water all over an unsuspecting sonographer? Drink two pints before your scan? Are they having a laugh? On a good day, most pregnant women can, at best, hold a thimble's worth of fluid before not being able to stand up straight and getting the wee sweats – that's before someone pummels you in the gut with an ultrasound machine.

With Jack, I remember lying in the darkened room, clenching for dear life, and waiting with bated breath as my internal organs were pressed harder than Bill Clinton at his impeachment. Finally, after what felt like a lifetime, amidst the whooshing black abyss on the screen, we saw him … a grainy black-and-white image of our unborn kidney bean. Bouncing off my uterine walls, flipping us the bird (a sign of what was to come), and with a strong little heartbeat pulsating with life. It was real. Tears slid down our faces – Steve's with pure and raw emotion, mine because I was about to wet myself.

Once the scan is out of the way, and hopefully the news is joyful and reassuring, you can take your grainy blob photos and cry in the car for half an hour. It's happening, it's actually happening. You are going to have to grow a human, and then somehow coax it out of your vagina as though it's a cat stuck up a tree. A lot of people choose to tell friends and family after the twelve-week mark, once they've seen that comforting and truly miraculous flutter of life, and statistically the threat of miscarriage is smaller. Unable to hold in secrets – or urine, in my case – Steve and I told both our families from around the six-week mark. What an awkward convo that is, by the way … admitting to your father that you've had a bit of, well, 'How's your father' (the weirdest expression, by the way). Given we were 27, both sets of parents *probably* knew it was a possibility we'd attempted a few of the bases, but it's still a fairly uncomfortable scenario for all concerned to confirm their suspicions of a home run. My dad's reaction to my first pregnancy was priceless. He shook Steve's hand and said, 'Well done' as though he'd just announced he'd passed his driving test, taking my L-plates along with him. He did have a little cry five minutes after, either with the emotion of it all or the realisation of where his son-in-law's hand had actually been. My biggest pet peeve when telling people your big news is when your partner announces to friends and family

'We're pregnant!' Hang on a minute, dickhead, are we? You got an orgasm and an early night, babes – come back to me when your insides have dislocated themselves like the jaws of a python about to swallow a pig.

I also found people's reactions to our big news to be a funny old thing. Some were delighted, some weren't even remotely bothered, and then there were those who couldn't wait to terrify the life straight out of me. It's the latter you need to watch out for because they'll send you into full-scale prenatal panic mode with talk of, a) how awful it is to be pregnant, b) how horrible children are, and c) how a gigantic, bodily-fluid-covered baby is going to head-butt its way out like a bull in a vag(ch)ina shop.

With the second trimester comes respite from some of the more debilitating pregnancy side effects, hurrah! Sickness begins to give way, your energy levels start to increase, and feelings of your old self may start to resurface … but in shittier clothes. Really annoyingly, and especially with your first baby, it takes quite a lot of time for your stomach to 'pop', resulting in a highly difficult 'has she stacked on weight, or is she pregnant?' no-woman's land. What this also means is that you aren't big enough for proper maternity clothes, but are too big for your normal clothes – stranding you in leggings and a jumper, regardless of the season. When you're finally big enough to fit into official maternity wear, there's only a couple of months left, and is there any point investing in elasticated denim? We all know once baby's out, your completely non-battered body just snaps back into its old form immediately (doesn't it?!) – so what's the point? In my second trimester, I also felt totally unsupported … because maternity bras are fucking shocking. One major high street retailer reduced me to floods of tears during a fitting because the lady touching me up with a tape measure discovered I was wearing a wire. Seriously, the mafia would have let me off more lightly than Marjory (circa 60 and with a highly scientific degree in 'raising her own children forty years ago') – who wasted no time in lecturing me about some horrific-sounding seventeenth-century boob rot, witchcraft, and a whole world of issues surrounding milk flow and blocked ducts. Apparently, my only options were hideously saggy and not sexy maternity bras that looked as though they belonged in a cobwebbed museum of chastity wear. The best bit about these over-sized, passion-destroying boulder holders was that they also doubled up as breastfeeding bras, complete with clippy bits that unhooked to reveal a sensual, highly engorged nip beneath. Steve was *very* excited when he first clapped eyes on them, thought I'd been to Agent Provocateur and treated him to some of those kinky peek-aboo numbers … until the time came to try them on, that was, and it became apparent they were much more peekaspew in nature.

It's not just your tits and tummy that expand throughout this trimester – your legs also decide to get in on the action by adopting the water storage capabilities of a camel. My knees were completely eradicated by this extreme stockpiling measure, along with my ankles, which blended seamlessly into the lower calve region, creating incredibly attractive cankles. Many an evening was spent alarmingly poking my legs and waiting to see how long it took for the finger indentations to disappear, and if Play-Doh legs weren't sexy enough, my feet also decided to completely let themselves go too, spreading like margarine on hot toast so that the only shoes my flat and fat hooves could get into were a pair of early noughties Ugg boots, or flip-flops. My poor libido also took a spanking too, and not in an S&M way, with the only screaming in the bedroom happening because of some seriously naughty leg cramps.

As well as some of the less enjoyable elements of this stage of pregnancy, some pretty amazing things also happen, such as being able to hear your baby's heartbeat at midwife appointments. A galloping horse, or runaway train? Could that be an indicator of the baby's sex? Steve and I decided we didn't want to know the sex of either of the kids – but that didn't stop me obsessively googling horse heartbeats, bump shapes, and Chinese prediction charts. Of course, there is one scientifically accurate way to find out – your twenty-week scan, another nail-biting milestone where you can indeed find out the flavour of your creation, and otherwise known as the foetal abnormality scan. This one caused me more worry than the twelve-weeker; it's a real hybrid of emotion – excitement at another chance to see your baby but there's also the shit-scary prospect of discovering a problem. With Evelyn's scan, we couldn't get a babysitter for Jack and so, with pre-scan anxiety levels already through the roof, we decided to up the ante by taking a hyperactive and highly vocal toddler with us. The situation was made all the more stressful by the fact he'd filled his nappy with the previous night's fish pie and of course we'd forgotten the change bag because we'd been parents for over twenty-four months and were still as disorganised as the moment he was born. While Steve incorrectly guessed she was a boy on the back of seeing what he proudly claimed to be a massive willy (otherwise known as an umbilical cord), there I was trying to stop a toddler from sticking his finger in wall sockets, and constantly apologising for the smell.

At some point between sixteen and twenty-four weeks there'll be the unmistakable and stomach-churning sensation of feeling your baby kick for the first time … or is it wind? The number of times I made Steve sit with his head on my bump, waiting for him to feel the tiny ripple of life from within, only to discover it was the spirit of the previous night's curry making its presence known … A few more weeks, however, and those butterfly flutters and pops of air suddenly turn into very definite and very real hoofs to the gut, ribcage, and bladder. Beautiful, magical …

vom-inducing. For me, it was when my pregnancies felt real. There was an actual person inside me that I could feel, talk to, fall in love with, and blame my questionable smells on. Beyond miraculous.

Once eased into the pregnancy journey, attentions may be turned towards what you might need to know prior to the arrival of the person responsible for all that wind. Pre-Jack, it's laughable how underprepared we were – something that became more apparent after the girls at work threw me a baby shower and I had a complete breakdown at seeing a pair of scratch mitts. Why would my baby try and claw me like an angry cat? Was that normal? This, combined with the fact I thought meconium was a type of metal, made me realise a more formal education in parenting, other than the internet, might not be a bad idea.

Attending NCT (Narky Childbirthers Together) classes was an eye-opener, and leg-closer – although it was arguably too late for that. Twenty minutes of watching a labour video that looked as though it should have been stored in a police evidence folder, the only thing I was prepared for ever coming out of me were red-hot tears of hysteria. 'I can't, Steve, I JUST CAN'T!' Held in one of the North West's finest working men's establishments, my group was an interesting collection of souls – trendy ones, older ones, younger ones, and of course overachieving ones, smugly clutching their copies of *What to Expect When You're Expecting*. Alright, knobheads, safe to say we've all done the sex ed homework. Sitting in a semi-circle with name labels peeling off us, glum faces, and stale biscuits, it was like being at a support group for those with DUIs as opposed to those with recently removed IUDs. Our fearless leader was a lovely lady named Jane who came bearing objectives, props, and a knitted placenta. My favourite part of the experience was roleplaying our lady gardens opening up into exquisite flowers, ready to birth our beautiful children into the waiting world. By that point, I hadn't seen mine in a while but was fairly certain it didn't resemble a bunch of geraniums and instead had changed colour, grown teeth and was much more reminiscent of a penis flytrap. After fifteen well-spent minutes passing round bottles of amniotic fluid, and a further thirty in the toilets scrubbing our hands, it was a hectic schedule of dressing dolls and dislocating their shoulders, identifying baby shit, translating the ancient language of crying, and a lovely little session where we wrote down all the nice things our partners could do for us after we'd given birth. Top of my list – a vasectomy.

Once you've semi-sussed how they're coming out, the second trimester is also when some consideration might go into deciding on what they're going to be called – aside from 'bump' or 'bean'. It's at this point massive falling-outs with significant others occur as negotiations over the highly political 'moniker' escalate. Any names of exes are completely off the cards, as are names of people you went to high school with and thought were dicks. Naughty kids of friends or neighbours are also out, as are dodgy names of family members entered on the 1801 census. At one point Steve and I had a cracking argument over the name Paula – I had nothing personal against it, apart from the fact we weren't living in the eighties and Paula Abdul was no longer that much of a big deal. It honestly felt as though we were going two steps forward, and one step back.

Thought also needs to go into all the stuff that has to be bought for them and how they're going to be transported to the pub and back. They need so many things – cots, Moses baskets, change units, wipeable mats, vests with a million different sleeve lengths, little bouncy chairs to throw up all over, cloths to wipe up said sick, sterilisers, dummies, and so on. The kid's yet to arrive and its rider is more demanding than Mariah Carey's.

Starting with the basics, we thought shopping for a pram would be a fairly easy first hurdle to overcome. Oh, how wrong we were. First off, they're not prams. No, they are 'travel systems'. Never mind wanting something that's lightweight and easy to maneuver – apparently you need incredibly high-tech transportation that wouldn't look out of place in a Transformers movie, and going on the price of them … most definitely a DeceptiCON. Some of them were more expensive than my car. ISOFIX? I didn't even know what that was, but was very much hoping it would repair the cavernous and haemorrhaging hole in my bank account. Up until very recently, the only times I'd heard the words 'rear facing' were in relation to sexual positions. According to the internet, it is in fact the safest way to travel in a car, and how my children would be travelling until they turned 18 – in a high-back booster with a five-point harness. Picking up first dates would be interesting – they for sure wouldn't get laid, but on the plus side if they got into an accident, their spines would be safe. It's not just the pram and the car seat, either. There are carrycots, footmuffs, sleeping bags, parasols and cup holders to think about. A word of advice here, just pick a pram/pushchair/thing with wheels that collapses without the need for a degree in mechanical engineering – there's not much worse than breast milk running down your legs in the Tesco carpark while you sweatily drop kick a £2000 broken pile of metal into the boot. There's so much choice; for many, it's totally overwhelming. My main criteria was that it matched my coat, but for Steve it was on a par with picking a new car. What about tyre treads? Does it have ABS brakes? And how does it handle on a wet road? Watching new dads in the park, proudly boasting about their new hot wheels' off-road abilities, complete with leather detailing and shiny alloys, is akin to watching an episode of 'Pop Gear'.

As a new parent, you get suckered into buying so many unnecessary items. *'No, I don't know what it does, Steve, but the baby magazine said I needed it, so we're buying it!'* Of course, I was a marketer's dream – a Tommee Tippee Perfect Prep that cost more than an espresso machine, despite plans to breastfeed; an anaconda-esque pillow to lay my nursing child on; baby CCTV everywhere so when they're crying at night they can be heard on monitors and turned down; mooing breast pumps to add that extra special dairy cow feeling. Hilariously, when it comes to your second child you don't bother digging all of the sacred first baby's shit-stained vests from out of the loft until a week before it's due. A new mattress? Absolutely not – they'll be alright on the dog's bed.

Your third trimester is when things start to heat up. Literally – sweaty pits, tits, and bits. Why is everything so hot, apart from your physical appearance? I'd had enough, the novelty had completely worn off, and literally no one had told me my vaginal lips would swell up as though they'd had pre *Love Island* filler. No knickers could contain them; I was worried I'd have to put out an amber alert in the North West for a wild big cat spotted in a heavily wooded area. I think it's safe to say that with both my pregnancies, from twenty-seven weeks onwards: not my finest moments. The 'ooh, you're all bump' comments were long gone and replaced with visible winces as my body entered its final metamorphosis from woman into *gut*terfly. Second time round was especially bad as my already stretched out stomach muscles, which all used to point in one direction, decided to go their own separate ways. With nothing holding back the baby, or the weight I'd gained from eating for two … hundred, the full girth of my belly was left to expand completely unrestricted. I'm talking gravitational pull of Jupiter massive, but instead of asteroids and space dust, I attracted elderly women in M&S who would ask if my twins were due soon. 'No, Edna, my one baby is due in ten weeks. Stop trying to touch my stomach. Now kindly fuck off.'

There was also a whole host of other late-pregnancy delights to contend with, one of which was itching. Oh, dear God, the itching. Boobs, belly, and some places that were less socially acceptable to scratch in public … that's right, if nature wasn't having enough of a laugh at my expanse, thrush was thrown in for good measure. Add in a need to pee approximately every fourteen minutes, back spasms, and a slowly separating pelvis that was causing me to walk like I'd gone at the yeast infection a little too hard – and I was feeling truly #blessed. Could I sleep for love nor money? Of course not, and if one more person told me 'it's just your body preparing for the baby arriving' I would have completely lost my shit. Although that's a lie, as I was also constipated. A far more logical way of approaching motherhood would be to allow pregnant women to get as much sleep as humanly possibly on the run-up to the impending birth so that by the time our babies arrive we're well rested, non-ratty, and less likely to put the baby down and not know where we've left it. Pillow talk, however, was at an all-time high … 'It's so big Steve, I can't wait for you to put it in between my legs … yes, that's it. Oh wow. It's so hard. Lovely, now can you fuck off to the spare room and leave me alone to spoon this four-foot-long maternity cushion. Thanks.'

With this trimester comes the most highly anticipated part of your pregnancy journey – the special moment you've been counting down the days to, and when it finally arrives it hardly seems real. MATERNITY LEAVE! Oh, it's the best feeling ever, waving goodbye to all those suckers in your office who don't have to go through a horrific amount of pain and then keep someone alive and out of jail for the next eighteen years. The lengths some people will go to just to get a bit of time off work. You can lie around eating cake, do some shopping, catch up on your favourite Netflix shows, have a prenatal pamper session, or go for lunch with your fellow knocked-up friends. Unless, that is, you already have children. In which case, scoffing half-eaten brioches, shopping for endless supplies of mini rice cakes, watching the same twelve episodes of *Hey Duggee*, scrubbing piss out of a carpet, and only eating in restaurants that serve food with a side of crayons is on the agenda.

During your final weeks of pregnancy, signs of nesting may start to materialise. Not normally known for my obsessively tidy ways, Steve thought I'd been replaced by bodysnatchers when he came home and found me hoovering the dog. Little did he know that it was actually the body in my snatch that was causing my newly acquired neuroses about hygiene. Very much in the same way your body starts mentally preparing for a sleep-free future, the third trimester starts preparing you for the dignity-free labour. Attempting to get 'baby-ready' but unable to see or reach my pregnancy bush, there was only one option and only one man for the job. Sitting on the toilet seat, safety goggles on, and brandishing his Gillette Mach3 in place of a Black+Decker hedge trimmer, my poor husband had to experience the very best a man could get … repetitive strain injury in his wrist. Took him nearly two hours to hack his way through it, and at one point I was absolutely convinced he'd taken off my clitoris.

Quite possibly one of the worst things to happen, however, was the perineal massage. If you don't know what this is, count yourself as one of the lucky ones. A preventative measure to reduce the likelihood of tearing or needing an episiotomy during labour, it basically involves stretching the skin between your vag and your ass, and was NOT what my husband had in mind when I asked if he'd like to try anal. Now, this can be done solo … but if reaching flowing locks of pubic hair is problematic, it's highly unlikely sticking a finger up your bum is going to be in your bag of party tricks. Jane from NCT made it sound so easy, almost romantic … a darkened room, a scented candle, Enya playing in the background … then 'pop' a thumb in and massage, until it burns, in the shape of a 'U' – presumably a 'FUCK U'. I should have known it was going to be a rough ride for us when I told him to get the peri oil and he walked in with a bottle of Nando's sauce. Definitely not the time for finger-licking deliciousness. Five minutes in, the only things stretched were the boundaries of our marriage.

In pregnancy, it's all about your due date – spending every waking minute counting down the days until finally saying hello to your bundle of joy and goodbye to an ability to sneeze without excessive clenching. The problem with due dates is that they are, annoyingly, incredibly inaccurate, with only 4 per cent of babies actually being born on the day they're supposed to be. Potentially more annoying than this is all the people who'll take great joy in gloating to you – now a fully fledged manatee – that first babies are always late.

By the time Jack's due date came and went, my body was falling apart – I'd had my fair share of pregnancy pitfalls and I could take no more. I'd tried convincing my body to engage in early-release negotiations with my cervix, to shave a bit of time off for good behaviour, but it was having none of it. So, what happens when your baby is so overdue someone has to call in the bailiffs? Mostly, a bombardment of unsolicited advice from people you know, and complete strangers, on 'how to get things going naturally'. Everyone, so it would seem, is an expert on how to get that baby out, and they are not beating around your bush. 'What about going for a hike?' Getting up just to go for a wee/trip to the fridge every five minutes was hard enough – I looked as though I was an extra in *The Walking Dead*. So no, a ten-mile walk with chub rub and the sensation of smuggling a bowling ball up my faff – not a great suggestion. People also seem to lose all sense of boundaries around heavily pregnant women. Random folk in supermarkets would say 'what about a little bit of …' then make an inappropriate whistling noise. What? Calling a cat in at night? Nope. Sex. It's a bit forward, isn't it? I'm also dubious about the science behind it, because if I was a small defenceless child and could see a one-eyed viper striking at me from the only exit point then I'd bloody well stay put too. There are many problems with this solution for both participants – the main being logistics. It is, however, one of these old wives' tales that – I'll begrudgingly admit – does seem to have an element of truth to it. After some googling on the subject (NEVER hit 'videos'), I found that lots of people claimed to have had great success. Here's the thing – money could be put on the fact that the only time your other half will lose their horn will be when you're forty weeks, covered in Dorito dust and crying because you no longer have knees. I didn't care if Steve thought 'doing the deed' would be the end of the world – at nearly two weeks overdue, I was ready for Acockalypse NOW!

'What about a really hot curry?' Another old wives' favourite. Have you ever eaten bowel-liquidising spiciness potentially twenty-four hours before putting a lot of effort into pushing a person out of your body? If you've failed at walking, bonking or shitting your baby out, you can always try bouncing it out. I spent days on a Swiss Ball, pounding the ground like Tigger on speed, and the only thing that came out of me was a bit of wee. The people said pineapple, which is my preferred fruit in a pina colada or on a pizza … but apparently it's the woody bit in the middle that needs to be gobbled down. Honestly, these old wives – monsters, every single one of them. My midwife, the only person actually qualified in the subject matter, suggested aromatherapy oils. She gave me a highly potent concoction called 'the bomb' to put in the bath … sounded promising … didn't go to plan. Not only did I not birth a baby, but this sea mammal had to suffer the indignity of being stranded in an oil slick. After downing four litres of raspberry leaf tea, the only thing left to try was ... the dreaded sweep. Over to a woman called Bev, with gloved hands the size of Shrek's, to spin out my cervix as though it was pizza dough. I could taste the latex – very much felt like she was trying to scratch my eyes out, from the inside.

I look back now at both of my pregnancy journeys with mixed emotions. There's a part of me that thinks 'thank God that's all over and done with' because, generally speaking, I was a fairly miserable host to my precious unborn cargo ... sicky, sweaty, and a savage in the company of carbohydrates. There is, however, also a part of me that's a teeny tiny bit sad our 'terrific twosome' adventures are over because it truly is the most indescribable, special, and humbling experience. It's also one of the most extreme physical and mental tests your body will go through – one that'll leave you exhausted, ill, emotional, scared and scarred. There were times my husband would look at me hurling in a bush, or bent double in agony with back spasms and would wish he could take it all away from me so I didn't have to go through it. Even if it were possible, à la Arnold Schwarzenegger in *Junior* (weirdest film EVER), I'd never let him because to me my pregnancies are badges of honour – privileges and not rights.

Each trimester was equally as 'trying', and every week felt painfully long, and even if you've had a complication-free journey, there's no such thing as an 'easy' pregnancy. Nine (nearly ten) months of ensuring the continuation of the human species is nothing to be sniffed at; it's one of the hardest jobs of all and is rewarded accordingly with the greatest gift of all ... a beautiful, precious, irreplaceable ... Gucci handbag. JOKES. Of course it's a baby ... of course it is ...

6

Miscourage

I'd being doing a disservice not only to myself, but to countless women if, on these pages, I didn't include a part of the pregnancy journey that isn't spoken about as much as conception, morning sickness, sneezy wees, or childbirth – and that is baby loss.

Now, here's your 'get out of jail free' card – if you'd like to skip this part then please proceed straight through to the next chapter. Maybe you've experienced loss yourself and it's still too raw to read about through someone else's eyes, or maybe you're worried it might make you feel a bit sad and that's not what you came here for. Either way, that's fine! There will never be any judgment from me. For those who'd like to stick around and read on, it's my hope, as always whenever speaking of this, to try and break down the unnecessary taboo surrounding miscarriage, hopefully empowering those who've been through it to talk more freely about their own experiences and for it not to feel like a shameful dirty secret to carry alone.

I've had the misfortune of experiencing early miscarriage twice, both ordeals differing from each other greatly. Very much like how two pregnancies are never the same, the process of losing them also varies massively. My first was between Jack and Evelyn – as you may recall, her arrival on this planet took a bit longer than her brother's due to a slight hold-up in obtaining planning permission from the powers that be. After what felt like endless trying, and probably hundreds of pounds spent on ovulation kits, imagine my excitement at realising my period was late and that FINALLY … the unsexy sex was over! It was so AWOL there was no doubt in my mind the result would be positive, so when test after test after test came back negative, I couldn't make head nor tail of it. I *had* to be pregnant – there was no other logical explanation … was there? Two weeks later, having upped my game and splashed out on a Clear Blue Digital test, eventually the positive result we were so desperately pining for arrived. Paying top dollar for something you urinate all over also came with the added bonus of telling me how many weeks I was, which would have been useful … apart from it wasn't. The pregnancy was only showing as being one to two weeks post-conception instead of the three plus it should have been, and no matter how many times I attempted to analyse my menstrual cycle and potential conception date, the numbers just didn't work out. Looking back, this warning sign was an ominous indication of what was to come. However, with no prior pregnancy problems to compare against, I put it down to a glitch in my cycle and carried on imaging how this new little person was going to seamlessly, and noisily, slot into our lives.

At around my six-week mark, Steve and I were about to go out with friends when an unsettled feeling in my stomach sent me legging it to the toilet. Norovirus had hit, and instead of a night on the tiles, I was vomiting on them. Concern struck me for two reasons, the first being that my pelvic floors weren't what they used to be, so with every heave the bladder walls gave way. Secondly, not one thing would stay down – so what did that mean for the ball of cells growing inside me? A panicked call to our GP eventually reassured me that the baby would be OK and as long as a few sips of water every now and again could be tolerated, we'd both be fine.

A few days later, thankfully feeling much better, Steve and I were snuggled on the sofa watching Ant and Dec do their thing on *I'm a Celebrity … Get Me Out of Here*, when I decided to go for my hundredth pregnancy wee of the hour. Standing up to go to the loo … it just happened. No warning, no pain, no indication that something was very wrong, until the very moment the warmth of blood seeped down into my underwear and soaked through to my leggings. It's funny how some days you can't even recall what you've had for breakfast, but when it comes to important or traumatic moments, those memories regularly replay in your mind, living vividly in 4K. Geordie accents blared from the TV in the background, while I emitted a piercing scream that didn't even sound remotely human. Running to the toilet shouting for Steve, I was utterly gripped by terror, and desperately hoping it wasn't as I'd feared and that I'd actually just wet myself. There was a phone call to 111, and a confusing conversation trying to quantify the amount of blood I'd lost through the medium of egg cups – all while I sat numbly on the toilet, my mind so paralysed with shock at the events unfolding that things weren't processing as they should. Having established there was no immediate danger, and that a hospital trip wasn't necessary – that's when the flood gates opened. Curled into the foetal position and wracked with sobs, pure heartbreak radiated through my body. Why was it happening to me? What did I do wrong? Willing that baby to hold on, the prospect of moving even the teeny tiniest amount was terrifying – convinced that even the smallest shift in my body weight would make it worse, and naively thinking gravity, along with fate, could be scuppered by my refusal to stand up.

Despite my Church of England education, religion wasn't something too high on my day-to-day agenda – but let me tell you ... it was that day. Prayers were said, along with promises to do charity work, solemn swears to buy *The Big Issue*, and vows to open the door to cold callers when they knocked – hell, I'd even invite them in for a cuppa. Here's what not do to if you ever find yourself in a similar situation: consult Dr Dread – aka Google – the only medical professional who can take you from a snotty nose to certain death in less than 0.0063 seconds. Flitting from pessimistic despair to unrealistic false hope, my head was a complete mess. Some webpages told me that bleeding in early pregnancy could be completely normal, others told me my baby's fate was sealed – but to be honest, in my heart of hearts and given the amount of blood lost, I knew nothing could have survived that. Despite this, it didn't stop me staying awake all night reading against-all-odds success stories, my howling sobs slowly diminishing into the whimpering sounds of a wounded animal as I drifted off into a restless and tormented sleep.

The next morning, we managed to get an appointment at our GP surgery, only to be told there was not really much they could do, which was fair enough, but it was the disconcerting lack of sympathy that irked me – it was though I'd turned up with a cold. They referred me to our local hospital's Early Pregnancy Unit (EPU); however, I couldn't be seen for another two days. TWO DAYS?! Going on how I was feeling at that precise moment in time, it felt like a life sentence. No, I simply needed to know right there and then what was happening, and to be done with the limbo of waiting, wondering ... driving myself crazy with delusions that everything might just be OK. Those two days didn't seem survivable. I completely shut down emotionally, refusing to tell my parents, sister, work, or friends. Jack was like a light in the dark. He helped me to function on a basic level, and gave me a reason to put one foot in front of the other. Whatever was going on mentally and physically had to be put on hold for bum-wiping, snacks, cuddles, feeding of ducks, and bedtime stories. I was so lucky to have him, and to have already had one successful pregnancy, when so many other women were going through exactly the same thing but didn't have that much-desired little person at home to dry my eyes and say 'I love you Mummy'. Steve tried his best to keep my spirits up, carefully trying to balance optimism with expectation. We both knew, realistically, that the pregnancy was over, but neither of us could bring ourselves to actually say the words out loud.

By the time we headed off to the hospital, my tears, as well as the bleeding, had lessened – I knew it was merely a matter of formality. At the EPU we were ushered into a room where bloods, urine and my history were taken, before being led into a dark room with a waiting sonographer. The poor woman was only doing her job, but in my mind she was the Grim Reaper – instead of a scythe in her hand, she was holding a transducer and a bottle of KY Jelly. The initial ultrasound couldn't find anything in my womb, apart from blood, so it was decided that an internal scan would be our best bet of locating such an early pregnancy. Sadly, it could not. As I was told my body had fully completed the miscarriage naturally, just one solitary tear fell from an eye, burning like acid as it slid down my face and onto the paper-coated bed beneath me. While we waited for a specialist midwife to come and talk to us, we were sent into the special 'sad' side-room no one ever wants to go in – depressingly stark with a box of Kleenex on the table, alongside a handful of leaflets on pregnancy loss. Sitting in silence on harsh blue plastic chairs, Steve and I gripped on to each other's hands, both not quite knowing what to say … me desperately wanting to get out of there and home to my baby so I could fully appreciate the miracle that was his life. The midwife arrived to inform me that my pregnancy hormones were next to non-existent, nature had done as it should and my body had successfully cleared everything itself – no further tests, results or explanation were required.

What I'd experienced was, apparently, 'very common' in early pregnancy. Those words cut me to the quick. Common? As in everyday, trivial, undistinguished? To me, it didn't feel common … it felt raw, painful, and unlike anything else I'd ever experienced up until that point in my life. To some it might have been a ball of cells, potentially yet to gain a heartbeat, but it felt as though I'd lost so much more … like a person's future had been ripped from my womb. I'd already imagined what those cells would grow into. If it was a boy, would he resemble Jack? How they'd fit into our lives, how the nursery would be redecorated … holidays as a four instead of a three, an extra Christmas stocking under the tree … The loss may have been medically 'run-of-the-mill' but for me it was a very real grief. Of course I projected blame onto myself … was it something I ate, or drank? Was it the stomach bug? Did I starve it of nutrients? Maybe being violently sick for two days, alongside all the stomach cramps, had loosened it from the lining of my womb … Ridiculous thoughts, but at the time, that's where my head was. Hundreds of questions raced through my mind, and I needed answers as to why this had happened. We left with none. At the time, early miscarriages in England weren't investigated until you'd suffered three concurrently. This policy of course has left millions of women none the wiser, wondering whether their losses could have been prevented, or whether they were indeed just 'one of those things'. We were sent home with a cheery parting note of 'I'm sure we'll be seeing you for a twelve-week scan with your next baby soon!' But I didn't want another baby, just the one that was gone.

I completely buried it, only telling a handful of people about what had actually happened, on a need-to-know basis. Forcing myself back into work just one week later, the stomach virus was a perfect cover-up for my absence. Slapping my make-up on like war paint, I fake-smiled my way through the days … a shell of myself, functioning just as much as was required. Despite initially being horrified at the prospect of trying for another baby, it transpired the only way for me personally to get past the trauma was to throw all of my efforts into trying to get pregnant again … to fill the empty void with another sense of purpose. There is a theory that, for whatever reason, your fertility is heightened after loss, and for us this seemed to be the case because only a couple of months later those two red lines popped up again. My pregnancy with Evelyn, however, was a totally different experience to carrying Jack – tainted by anxiety and fear, every trip to the toilet expecting to see blood-filled underwear, every little twinge catastrophised into the beginning of the end. I was a complete nervous wreck until the twenty-week scan, when all of her test results came back as normal. The trauma had been swapped for the joy I felt when she finally arrived, and so I continued on with life foolishly believing all my grief had been appropriately dealt with. It wasn't until the summer of 2020 that I realised it most definitely hadn't.

It was August, Covid-19 was running riot, and England was just about coming out of the grip of another national lockdown. Standing in my bedroom and holding on to one of my boobs, having just whacked it with a hairbrush, a shooting pain radiated from the nipple all the way through to my ribcage. Although a bit unusual for me, I chalked it up as a premenstrual warning sign because a pregnancy wasn't on the agenda AT ALL. We already had two children, and although having campaigned strongly for a third baby only a year earlier, it was something we'd both agreed to put to bed. Knee-deep in a pandemic, it was not an ideal time to expand the family – I had no desire to be trapped inside with my husband, cabin-crazy kids, and a newborn. Checking my phone to see when my period was due, it was a relief to see Aunt Flo was only a few days away – nicely explaining away the boob ache. At least there'd be a valid reason to don the chin-high granny pants, and impose a strict two-metre 'no touching' social distancing rule with my husband. It's funny how when you're in your twenties, the prospect of your monthly period seems like such a sexual inconvenience – whereas in your thirties, with a couple of sprogs, it's considered a week off that NO ONE is taking away from you.

Seven days later. Still no period. Panic had set in. The boobs were definitely more sore, and bigger – looking down at the them, it was as though Phil and Grant Mitchell had taken up residence in my bra. Having sent an SOS (Stressed Out Sophie) to Steve, he'd returned home from work with the cheapest pregnancy test he could find and six bags of Kettle Chips because they were on offer for £1. False fucking economy, Steve, because regardless of the result, guess who's being sent out to get the idiot-proof digital one AS PER INSTRUCTIONS. In the bathroom, with kids banging on the door on what was the hottest day of the year, I tried to squeeze out a solo drop of dehydrated wee – my patience was as worn as the crotch of my baggy leggings.

'Leave me alone, Mummy's on the toilet!!' I spat at my snack-craving children, with the wrath of a sweaty and unacclimatised hell demon.

'Sorry, are you going to be long?' A nervous voice trembled through the door. Not the children, but Dave, my builder who was midway through our kitchen extension. Escaping the bathroom, past a doubled-over middle-aged man, and having sought refuge in my bedroom, I slammed the door and slid down against it, mentally preparing to await my fate. It wasn't possible … was it? We'd been careful … hadn't we? No, there was no way …

Pregnant.

I'm still a tiny bit ashamed to say tears fell from my eyes, and not the happy ones. Even though I'd been the biggest champion of another child for a fair while, this was different because it wasn't planned. Things were also moving forwards for me career-wise, plus the previously mentioned novel virus ravaging the planet. It just felt like the worst timing in the world. Steve actually took it better than me, despite always being strongly in the 'no' camp for a third, which really surprised me. After finally getting my head around it, at circa seven weeks, a problem arose. Spotting. There wasn't a lot of blood but enough to spark a little voice of anxiety in my mind that told me something wasn't right. Dr Google (I never learn) told me this could be perfectly normal during early pregnancy – it was dark and nothing like the torrent of blood from my first experience, which made me feel better – but still, I was uneasy. This time, not bothering with the GP, a phone call was made directly to a community midwife who listened intently while I relayed my fears. Because of Covid, reassurance scans at EPUs weren't allowed, but as I'd had bleeding and a previous miscarriage she managed to arrange a referral for the next day, which was a huge relief. Do you know what? I didn't feel like there was a serious problem at that point, mainly because the bleeding was minor in comparison to what had happened a few years earlier. If I'm being honest, I was fretting more about the prospect of there potentially being more than one in there … Twins.

Steve wasn't allowed to come with me – Covid restrictions wouldn't allow it – so he stayed at home with the kids and I drove myself to the hospital. Not quite sure what to expect, but still not actually expecting the worst, it wasn't until I was lying on the bed busting for a wee in the ultrasound room, the lights dimmed, that things hit home. The look on the sonographer's face gave everything away. 'How many weeks are you?' she asked, while gliding her equipment over my stomach.

'Seven' I replied, nervously, my voice squeaky with a sudden wave of fear.

'OK' she said, turning her screen to face me. 'What I'm looking at here is a much earlier pregnancy, possibly about four to five weeks.' And there, on the monitor, quite clearly in the darkness of my own uterus was a glowing white orb … but it was completely empty. Reading my panicked expression, she tried to bolster my spirits by explaining my dates were more than likely off and things probably just weren't as far along as I'd thought. But my dates were correct, this I was certain of – as a busy mum of two who'd been married upwards of ten years, opportunities for conception aren't exactly plentiful. Something was not right.

On my own, with tears sliding down my face as the internal wand was used to confirm what the external scan was showing, the heart-wrenching realisation it had happened again washed over me. This time, however, there was no one to hold my hand, to tell me everything was going to be OK, and no one to ask the questions my shell-shocked brain was incapable of asking. Afterwards, it was a trip back to the same sad waiting room I'd experienced nearly six years prior, every single detail of it as clear in my mind as though it were the day previous. A midwife informed me the scan was inconclusive. There was no heartbeat and normally by seven weeks there is; however, it's not a given, which is why they'd have to leave it another two weeks before they could make the call on whether it was a missed miscarriage or not. Up until that moment, I'd never heard of such a term. A missed miscarriage? Apparently also known as a silent miscarriage – when an embryo has not developed or has died but there are no typical symptoms such as bleeding or cramping. Sent away, it was now a waiting game … either the pregnancy would progress, or I'd miscarry. With the weight of the world on my shoulders, the solo walk back through the hospital to the car park was tortuous. Tears streamed down my face, pooling in my facemask, as people looked at me with a mix of sympathy and alarm. The hospital was heaving, and fury grew inside me – why was it fine for all these people to be there when I'd just gone through one of the most traumatic hours of my life without anyone to support me? The injustice burnt deep from within my chest. Climbing back into the car, a tidal wave of emotion crashed out of me, and by the time I called Steve I was completely incomprehensible through the snot, tears, and gulps of breath.

The following weeks were horrendous; it was the worst form of limbo. Constantly on my phone calendar trying to convince myself maybe I'd got the dates wrong. Googling the lifespan of sperm, then trying to make research fit with my own false-hope-filled agenda. By the end of the first week I'd nearly booked myself in for a private scan because I felt so unable to tolerate the misery of waiting to miscarry any longer. When might it happen? What if it was in front of the kids, or in the middle of a supermarket? I was too scared to even go for a walk. A midwife friend convinced me to stick it out and wait for the hospital appointment, otherwise I'd be wasting money and mental reserves just be told the same – the two weeks were vital for a conclusive answer. Patience was a virtue, apparently.

This time round I did, however, decide to tell people what was happening … my parents, in-laws, sister and some select friends. My network of fellow mums were all amazing, taking it in turns to doorstep me supplies of chocolates and flowers, and send me messages – they even attempted to prise me out of the confines of my four walls. It was amazing how much difference talking about it actually made, though. My load felt instantly lightened.

It transpired at least three of my close friends had been through similar experiences of missed miscarriage. When asked why they hadn't said anything, they all pretty much replied with the same … they didn't want to tell people because they felt like they couldn't, it was too socially awkward, or they felt they were burdening others with their grief. What do you say to someone when they tell you they might lose or have lost their baby? I get it, it's uncomfortable and not the type of conversation you'd have with someone down at your local Tesco. But us women do this strange thing when we find out we're pregnant – we don't tell anyone … we keep it a big secret, fundamentally because the fear of something going wrong and then having to upset people with the bad news is too much to bear. In reality, it's the people closest to us we need the most when things don't go to plan – by not telling them, how are they supposed to help us when things do take a turn for the worst? There's also an odd underlying level of shame associated with miscarriage; it's a taboo subject that's not spoken about enough – totally baffling, considering it affects one in four women. We feel as though we did something wrong, we're unfit to be mothers, not worthy of the life that should be growing within in us. In most cases we're only guilty of falling victim to nature, to odds, to a miscalculated cell divide. Thinking about it, given the low odds of sperm actually meeting egg, in any given month, on top of the potentially plentiful list of things that could go wrong in the early stages post-fertilisation, it's miraculous human beings are still here.

Finally, my two weeks were up and it was time for the follow-up scan. I'd had no further bleeds, my boobs were continuing to expand – as was my waist (third baby and your abdominal wall gives up the ghost pretty early). There were cravings, bouts of nausea, and extreme tiredness. On paper, this was a normal pregnancy that was progressing. I had begun to wonder if I'd actually made life worse for myself by going for the early scan

– might all of this worry and upset have been for nothing? Another kick in the teeth, especially given that at the time Boris Johnson had launched the 'Eat Out to Help Out' scheme encouraging the whole of the UK to get back out there and spread some germs around in the interests of boosting the economy, was that Steve could still not come with me for the appointment. Despite there being a very strong chance bad news was on the horizon, I'd still have to fly solo. At this point, though, my emotions felt a little bit more stable – I just needed to know, and for it to be over. It was either happening, or it wasn't.

Lying on the bed, I was steeled for the sympathetic hand-stroke and bad news I'd been anticipating, so when I heard the word 'progression' leave the sonographer's mouth, it seriously did not release the hope and happiness you might have expected, but confusion and pure panic. There within the floating white orb was a microscopic little dot, apparently a tiny foetal pole that was not visible at the last scan. Most ominously, and notably missing, however, was any trace of a heartbeat. Now, I'd had a reassurance scan with Evelyn at just six weeks and saw her fast-beating flicker of life immediately, so I knew that by nearly ten weeks there should have been more than a ghostly floating ball. But there was nothing. The problem here, however, was the word 'progression'. The egg sac had grown, and because they could now see an indication of potential life in the form of the pole (arguably missed first time), the hospital was unable to morally make the call – they had to give it one final week to see if a heartbeat developed. In my mind, this was absolutely devastating. It was just not possible for it to be a viable pregnancy – my first dating scan was in a couple of weeks and there I'd be expecting to see something that vaguely resembled a jumping kidney-bean-shaped baby – not an empty, lifeless blob. It was also an unimaginable horror, the prospect of having to go away for another week and relive the same mental hell as the previous fortnight. I was now also filled with a scenario I'd yet to fully contemplate – what if this pregnancy continued, but there was a severely life-limiting problem with the baby growing inside me? My dates were accurate, and for the embryo to be developing so slowly without a heartbeat terrified me more than the prospect of losing the pregnancy. This was not a child thriving in the safety of my womb, so in my mind there was very little possibility of it flourishing outside.

Seven days of mental anguish passed, still with no sign of my body giving up its precious cargo. Steve drove me back to the hospital and again waited in the car park as I headed in for what would hopefully be my third and final scan. It was. At eleven weeks, there had been no change, no further growth, and no heartbeat. Salty tears poured from my eyes, but this time they were mostly laced with relief … It was finally over, and now something could be done. It was never a real baby, it didn't ever truly live, and although grieving the loss and notion of what could have been, I also needed to move on with my life and concentrate on my babies at home who'd had a pretty awful and emotionally detached mummy for the best part of a month. The scan showed there were already traces of bleeding in my womb, signs that my body was eventually beginning to catch up to the situation – it was finally doing as it should have done weeks ago. Looking back, one of my residual feelings over what happened is anger … anger that I didn't know what was happening, that my body tricked me into feeling and believing in a pregnancy that never truly was. There was no life to support, yet it fooled me into feeling like there was for weeks and weeks. The boobs, the sickness, the tiredness – it was a big con.

The hospital recommended medical management; it was the fastest method and given the pandemic, it wouldn't require an overnight stay. On being led out of the ultrasound room and back into the waiting room, I was faced by a lady waiting to go in after me. Perfectly put together, immaculate hair and make-up, a smart two-piece – but also alone, her eyes filled with absolute terror. Later, while sitting on the gynaecology day ward, the same woman was brought to the bay opposite me and before the curtains closed around her, I caught a glimpse of her eyes again – surrounded by smudged make-up. She was no longer perfectly put together, but shattered into a million pieces. It's an image that still haunts me to this day.

The process of inducing the miscarriage was worse than I'd imagined. Internal pessaries were used to kick things off, which felt like a further violation after all the poking and prodding I'd already endured. I had to stay on the ward for an hour or so afterwards, to ensure there was no reaction to the medication, before being discharged to miscarry at home. The ferociousness with which my body expelled the 'products of conception' completely caught me off-guard. It was nothing like the relatively pain-free loss I'd experienced first time. There had been a forewarning about the bleeding and what to expect when I passed the sac – but I wasn't quite expecting the immense pain and labour-like contractions that codeine and paracetamol failed to touch. A large bleed landed me back in hospital only a couple of hours later, but fortunately, thanks to an amazing senior nurse, this time Steve was allowed to stay. I didn't catch her name but if she ever happens to read this, thank you from the bottom of my heart. Her act of kindness and refusal to let a woman she'd never met miscarry on her own in the waiting room of a busy A&E department means more than I'll ever be able to express in words.

The aftermath was upsetting, confusing, angering, relieving, emotional, and extremely difficult. Cruelly, the lingering hormones plagued me for weeks, my sore and swollen breasts mocking me at every opportunity, random nausea, and a superhuman ability to smell things from miles out reminding me of what I no longer was. Feelings I'd suppressed from my first miscarriage resurfaced; it felt like the worst BOGOF ever. I did, however, have an amazing support network, and even though social distancing was in place, my friends and family went out of their way to look after me. This time around, I was self-employed so was under no pressure to get myself back to work. A job in comedy doesn't lend itself well to recovering from a traumatic event – and it really is a trauma, you know, and a grief. If you are going through this, or have been through it, take some time to be kind to yourself – for your body, and mind. Removing myself from social media helped to eradicate the additional noise … took me away from pictures of happy couples announcing pregnancies, or cradling newborn babies – it wasn't something I needed in my life. On making the decision to rejoin the online world, I hesitantly decided to use the platforms to talk about my journey – not only for myself (although incredibly cathartic) but for others who'd also been down the same long and painful road. Stifled by society's discomfort at speaking of baby loss, thousands of messages from both men and women flooded my inboxes. I was even stopped in the park, walking the dog, by a total stranger who wanted to talk about his own experience. How wonderful that two complete strangers could have such a frank and honest conversation with one another about such a difficult topic. It was validation that raising the issue and speaking out was really the right thing to do – after all, a problem shared is a problem halved. Sometimes it's much easier to share painful words with people you don't know – especially the ones who have been through the same struggle – and know what to say in return. Us Brits are known for our stiff upper lip, our ability to crack on with things instead of cracking in the face of emotion. We shy away from miscarriage because it makes us feel awkward AF, but if it were to be discussed more freely maybe it wouldn't feel so alien to us?

I quite often get asked for advice on how to get over a miscarriage. The truth is that I don't think it's ever something you can truly forget or get over; life does carry on, though, and although a cliché, time really is a great healer. I kept the positive pee sticks (gross, I know) from both miscarriages – I like to look at them every now and then as proof that, if only for a short time, they existed in this world. Talking really does help too – family, friends, a stranger on the internet or in the park, a support worker at the end of the phone. If you feel ready, and comfortable, it can really make the world of difference. I'm now very philosophical about my own journey. I quite often stare at Evelyn in awe – she's incredible, one of the best humans imaginable and full of such spirit, imagination, and sass – I feel truly humbled to be her mummy. She wouldn't be here if the first miscarriage hadn't happened, and I know I'd feel the same way about the baby that never was, but I just can't imagine a world without my daughter in it – so for that, I am appreciative.

My advice to those wanting to support someone going through miscarriage would be to take their lead, and just be a listening ear. Don't force them to talk if they aren't ready; send messages to let them know you are thinking of them and you're ready and waiting when they're ready to open up. Drop a meal on a doorstep, offer to look after their kid/dog/partner for the day. I know you won't mean to offend, and it'll come from a place of love, but try to avoid saying things like 'it's so common', or 'you'll be able to get pregnant again' – although imparted with good intentions, those well-versed phrases can trivialise a person's feeling of loss.

Thank you so much for sticking with me throughout this difficult chapter; it was as hard to write as it probably was to read. Never forget, no matter your situation in life – the ups, the downs, the heartbreak – we are all blooming miracles! So appreciate yourself, your loved ones, and your babies (even the ones you didn't get to hold).

7

Planet Birth

Chances are if you're female, yet to have children, and possess ears, you'll have probably heard several labour horror stories that will have left you screaming 'AN EPISIWHATOMY?!' You see, women with prior experience in the birthing battle arena are like bears – they have a great knack of sniffing out fearful and fresh meat ripe for the scaring. 'This one's menstruating – get her!' As a semi-experienced mother figure, honestly, this kind of outrageous and scaremongering behaviour is … hours of fun.

Yes, birth – the final front-bottom-tier. Let me just tell you … nothing will ever prepare you for the actual event of bringing life into this world. Not a book, not an NCT class, and not an unrealistic Hollywood movie … although, truth be told, Alien *might be a fairer representation than most.*

Now, I've done this act of sheer madness twice, to date, so you're probably thinking 'well, it can't have been that bad if she went back for more!' Well, it was, but here's the thing about Mother/ Brother Nature – she's a bitch. How it happened, I'm not entirely sure … witchcraft, trickery, a cracking deal on duty-free rum … But a year or so after having Jack, somehow the entire shit show of my first birth was erased from memory, like a scene out of *The* Born *Identity*, and all too soon I was back to cooing over teeny tiny potato babies in public parks. What a con artist! Cunning, devious, manipulative, nature uses hormones to dupe the parts of our brains responsible for self-preservation, specifically the bit that goes 'Wait! That hurt like hell last time, best not do it again!' Girls, the biggest lie we will ever tell ourselves is that childbirth wasn't *that* painful. It's *even* worse than when you tell yourself it's fine to eat a whole bag of Mini Eggs because later you'll eat an apple and do six sit-ups. Despite being completely done over last time – left bleeding and needing stitches – the pain, indignity, and ordeal of it all oddly dissipates into nothing but a blurry recollection of it being a *'bit uncomfortable'*. UNCOMFORTABLE?! It's not trapped wind! It's a trapped human and they're clawing their way out by all means necessary. Why do all other traumatising life memories remain, while the horror of childbirth fades faster than a cheap box-dye? I'll tell you: because the human race depends on us females being able to hit the factory-reset button on the rational side of our psyche, completely forgetting the atrocities in favour of the continual population of the species. It's a little phenomenon I like to refer to as:

babynesia
Pronunciation: /beɪbiˈniːzɪə/
NOUN
[MASS NOUN]

A partial or total loss of memory that occurs after the horror of childbirth

Daft cow's pregnant again – she must be clinically insane or suffering from a severe case of babynesia.

A great example of this anomaly is my daughter's existence on these earthly plains. She's absolutely immense, and I aspire to be just like her – a ballsy, confident, assertive, princess-dress-wearing, Nerf-Gun-toting firecracker. A world without her in it would be a far less joyful and colourful place to exist. That said, the residual trauma left behind by the arrival of her brother years earlier had initially made me adamant he was going to be an only child – that was until babynesia kicked in … then I turned into Dory from *Finding Nemo*, wanting my husband's sperm to 'just keep swimming, just keep swimming'. The reason behind the initial reluctance was down to Jack's birth being so very, very difficult. At the point of marrying Steve, I had no idea all the boys born to his side of the family came out the size of Dwayne 'The Rock' Johnson – like they'd all been downing protein shakes and shoulder-pressing livestock from the moment of conception. I can't stress enough how very important it is to quiz any potential suitor, BEFORE committing to a life with them, whether their birth made it into the *Daily Mail*. Make informed decisions, people. Now, I didn't realise I was growing a boy, or that he'd be big enough to go on all the good rides at

Alton Towers from the age of one, but the very fact that at five months pregnant I resembled an anaconda that'd swallowed a horse, it really should have been a good indication. It's worth noting that a big baby doesn't necessarily equal a difficult birth – for me there were a number of issues that combined to make things trickier than any of us had expected …

There's a well-known military expression that 'proper prior planning prevents piss-poor performance', *unless* you're giving birth that is … then preparation goes out of the window faster than a grounded teenager sneaking off to a nightclub. When it comes to labour, even the best 'you got laid' plans have a slight tendency to go awry. With Jack, my plan mostly consisted of pushing him out of my vagina and taking all the drugs I was legally entitled to, an ambition realised by a very wise midwife who informed me you didn't get a medal on the way out of the labour ward for being a hero. That, my friends, was all the incentive required to BRING ON THE PARTY! On a serious note, there's no shame in taking the drugs – it doesn't make you any less of a mother because you didn't particularly enjoy the sensation of being torn in half. We're all made differently, with different pain thresholds – you just do you, babes! You probably know someone who did it on the love of a heavily bearded partner and pixie dust – but it's your experience so if you want to get tanked on prescribed narcotics, go for it. No judgement here.

Twelve days overdue, and after a sketchy moment of not being able to detect a foetal heartbeat, the decision was made to induce me. You know that scene in *The Exorcist* when the girl's lying on the bed and her head spins round 360 degrees? Welcome to my birthing video! Wow. The pain went from 0 to 100 in a *very* short time. When Steve suggested trying a slightly more natural approach of a TENS machine before heading straight for the heavy-duty drugs, I suggested strapping his penis to an electrical circuit at the same time so we could compare notes. If you're not the one having a baby, then FUCKING SHUT YOUR DAMN DIRTY PIE HOLE. No one cares about your opinion. Come back to me after trying to push an 8 lb-plus tricky poo out of the wrong hole, then we'll talk. Embodying the spirit of a true Brit at an all-you-can-eat breakfast buffet, this Scouse girl decided to go balls-deep – trying a little bit of everything, before going back for seconds. Gas and air, aka 'laughing gas', needs an advertising standards review, by the way – didn't chuckle once … too busy chucking up over several hard-working members of the NHS. Apologies to them. Diamorphine sent me OFF MY NUT – I lost several hours of my life and have a very vague recollection of attempting to hit on said vomit-covered NHS staff. 'You have very pretty eyes, but I do not like the smell of your perfume. Call me.' Again, apologies. I'm also fairly certain the International Space Station was able to transmit my high-frequency screams for an epidural from 220 miles above the earth. To be honest, I'd expected it to hurt – after all, it's called 'labour' – but I was *totally* unprepared for the intensity and longevity of it … or the mooing noises. Nobody tells you that the 'transition' phase involves you turning into cattle.

After almost forty hours in labour, thrashing around like a mating whale, with a back-to-back baby and my cervix stuck at 9 cm, my hopes of a natural birth were fading faster than my chances of ever again being able to wear a triangle bikini. The room gradually filled with more and more medical staff; 20-year-old Disney-prince-esque doctors were rummaging around in my nether regions like they'd lost their Rolex while I gave them my best 'come to my bed … AND GET THIS BLOODY BABY OUT!' eyes. Hushed discussions were being held in corners, while monitors were under constant review, until eventually the decision about how my baby was to be born was out of my hands … and sadly not out of my vagina. Turns out, much like me on a night out, the only way Jack was leaving was to be forcibly removed with brute strength. But wait, a Caesarean section was not in my birth plan! I'd signed myself up for a natural (drugs aside) birth – where he'd emerge from my nether regions and be presented to us like a scene out of *The Lion King*. The pair of us really hadn't discussed what would happen in the eventuality of me being rushed to theatre, and as a result, what followed next came as a very unwelcome bolt out of the blue. My epidural had apparently been sited incorrectly, numbing only one side of my body, so when it came to the slicing and dicing element of the extraction, I could still feel *EVERYTHING*. The absolute horror. Didn't cover that in NCT, did they? Thanks for the knitted placenta, Jane, but you forgot to mention the bit about your birth becoming part of the *Saw* movie franchise!

With no time to correct it or offer me a spinal, the only option was for a general anaesthetic. Steve had been an uncrackable and stoic fortress of emotion – keeping his panic levels calmly bubbling just below the surface – but as they ushered him out of the room fear flashed through his eyes, and well … I completely lost it. Hysterical and petrified, my arms were stretched out and strapped down, a foul-tasting liquid was poured down my throat and hands pushed onto my neck to make sure it'd been swallowed. Took me right back to my university sambuca days. It was as though everything was in slow motion, but also in fast forward at the same time … Medical professionals were blurred streaks of blue as they darted around the theatre, metallic clangs of surgical equipment rung in my ears, and as the room went black my final thoughts were 'please don't let my baby die …'

Whether it was God repaying me for a previous good deed (unlikely), or I'd made a half-lucid deal with the devil (more likely), when my eyes finally reopened, there was Steve … baby in arms, the fear in his red and puffy eyes replaced with relief and pure joy.

'It's a boy!' he gushed. Still half off my face, and mostly still cow, communicating emotion or sound in any form other than a groggy 'mooooooooooo' was difficult.

'Guess how much he weighed? He's 10 lb 10 oz!'

'YOU FUCKING WHAT?!' That woke me right up, didn't it? No chuffing wonder I couldn't get him out of me – my cervix hadn't been able to expand to the diameter of a megalodon's gob. Thank God it didn't, though … would have been like a black hole opening up, the whole world being sucked into the gravitational force of my collapsing faff.

There's no easy way of birthing a baby, is there? Vaginal or Caesarean, whichever way your child enters the world, it can be a deeply traumatic experience. I've had friends whose births have been longer and more difficult than mine and friends who've nearly birthed their babies in hospital car parks – fast labours seemingly no better than their marathon counterparts. What's apparent is not only the physical scars they leave behind, but also the mental ones. Undeniably, your body has just been through a feat of superhuman proportions, so why is it we're not more rewarding of ourselves and the pretty amazing job we've done?

In the weeks and months after his arrival, there was a definite mental struggle for me in terms of how things went down … I'd been totally robbed of my planned birth experience, and it left me feeling internally bereft. Poor Jack, it was as though neither of us were there when he finally made his appearance … Daddy was nowhere to be seen, and Mummy was conked out from drugs – hopefully not a premonition as to how the rest of his life would unfold.

Daydreams about what it'd be like laying eyes on my baby for the first time had vanished; there was no *Lion King* moment of seeing him held out in front of me – giraffes bowing down to us and monkeys flinging their shit around. It was emotionally devastating, and left me feeling bitter. Why didn't I get the same moment so many other women had? Programmes like *One Born Every Minute* were unceremoniously deleted from the TV amidst my refusal to see or hear of other people having their perfect births. Retrospectively, this now seems utterly ridiculous – because the universe gave me a perfectly healthy baby boy, and everyone survived. The fact it was a C-section when we'd planned for a 'natural' birth, in all honesty, hugely impacted on my post-partum journey. It gnawed away at my soul that I didn't do it 'properly', that I'd failed at something the female body, in theory, was designed to do. You read about the negative associations connected to Caesareans all the time – you're 'too posh to push', or you've taken the 'easy way out' … out of where? Alcatraz? Half-naked, strapped to an operating table that's too narrow for your chubby Mars-bar-loving arse, all while MASSIVELY regretting letting your other half hack at your bush with a semi-blunt Gillette. At that moment in time you are not posh, privileged, lazy or living your best life – you're cut in half, shit-scared, and sporting a very questionable muff mohawk. The word 'natural' would cut me as deep as the scalpel that carved out my presumably 'unnatural' birth – especially when expressed by judgemental types who thought they deserved a badge of honour for delivering their children via their birth canal, and not through their 'guilt canal'.

'Oh, did you not *manage* it naturally?' Always said with a condescending head tilt. Nope … and if I had, then my cavernous, galaxy-destroying, bone-splicing vagina would have swallowed us all whole so … YOU'RE WELCOME.

Because of my C-section hang-ups, when babynesia struck and gifted me Evelyn, in my mind there was absolutely no way another 'slice and dice' delivery would be taking place. The kid was coming out of the main exit whether she liked it or not: hello the VBAC (sounds like a nineties boyband, but actually stands for Vaginal Birth After Caesarean). Something not really contemplated in my decision-making process was that maybe I'd just not been designed for birthing babies – an issue that became much more apparent the second time round. If prior access to a crystal ball had been available showing my five-year-old daughter to be a highly stubborn, unpredictable, anti-establishment rebel, I'd have re-evaluated trying to push her into a dark hole. You see, Evelyn doesn't do *anything* she doesn't want to, and she most certainly did NOT want to go gynaecological potholing. Despite her arrival in this world a week earlier than planned, she was happy to be intravenously fed cake and wasn't prepared to leave my womb without a big fuck-off fight.

Again, we chose not to find out the sex but were told that if 'for example' it was a girl then she'd likely be smaller and so stood a better chance of exiting via the front door instead of the sunroof. An early sweep was booked for thirty-eight weeks, to see if we could get things going – if that failed then I'd be induced on my due date.

About two days after my sweep, something was birthed … sadly it was less 'squishy baby you wanted to snug', and more 'squishy blob that looked like a slug'. Scooping it up and shoving it under Steve's nose, I was like, 'BABE!! WHAT IS THIS?! Oh wait … don't worry – think it's just my mucus plug!', delighted, of course, as he dry-heaved into the bathroom bin, because it meant *something* was happening. The following day, while leaning over the bath with Jack, fluid gushed down my legs … this was it! First my plug, then my waters – it was go-time! After dragging Steve out of the pub, rushing to the hospital, then sitting in the maternity unit for three hours – we were home. Turns out, I'd just pissed myself. Awkward. The following days were a nightmare; contractions came and went – as did I, from the hospital. With a VBAC, the minute you get a hint of labour you have to be assessed because of the possible risks of scar rupture. On three separate occasions we were told the baby would be arriving that day, only to be sent home hours later because my contractions had completely disappeared. Transpires Evelyn didn't get the memo that babies are meant to come out of 'V's, not flip them. Five days later, and having ugly-cried in the maternity unit, a kind-hearted midwife took pity on me and managed to break my waters – finally kicking off my active labour and absolutely annihilating my new slippers. Here's a word of advice when packing your hospital bag – don't bother getting yourself fancy new birthing slippers, or new birthing anything for that matter. Grab something your dog has already slept on and partially shredded – the addition of extra bodily fluids won't make a difference and you'll be happy to burn it on a ceremonial bonfire afterwards, while repeatedly chanting the sacred words 'never again, never again, never again, never again'.

Before my first birth, my Google searches consisted of '*How* do you know if you're in labour?' HA! I've since discovered it's fairly easy: if you're spitting venom like a cornered cobra, and threatening to shiv a midwife with a catheter, you're in labour. The minute my waters went and my daughter's bony little head ground into my unyielding cervix, the babynesia fog ironically lifted and it dawned on me with face-slapping clarity how painful labour was … I was like a furious Celine Dion, 'IT'S ALL FUCKING COMING BACK TO ME NOW! GIVE ME THE SECTION!'

In a bid to do things differently this time, I'd decided that in order to open my cervix, first I must open my mind … with holistic approaches to birthing. Levelling with you, birthing pools – not my bag. Didn't much fancy stewing in a slow cooker of my own juices and floating excrement. '*Pass the sieve, Steve!*' However, if it meant getting the baby out non-surgically, a sacrifice could be made. I lasted all of about twenty-five minutes. The natural way could knob off. I wanted it all – an aerial assault team dropping in from the ceiling with epidurals, nineties It girls strutting in with lines of powder and syringes of whatever they could find on the street corner. At one point, a doctor offered me liquid paracetamol while we waited for the anaesthetist. *'I'm sorry ... CALPOL?!'* Bitches be cray. Eventually someone arrived with injectable narcotics that weren't strawberry flavoured, and the world once more became a better place. Shortly after, the epidural arrived and the prospect of being able to push a baby out became feasible again. Well, so I thought. Hours passed and nothing seemed to be happening, apart from Steve's incessant need to continually pet me like a cat. Labouring cats especially do not enjoy being touched. A lesson he, and his hand, learnt the hard way. My cervix had reached the much-coveted 10 cm dilation marker, though – but a baby hadn't fallen out, and no one was telling me to push. There was also a problem brewing ... in my gut. A number two was most definitely on the horizon, and not the second-child variety. Excuse the pun here, but this was pooh-poohed by the medical team – apparently it was just my body telling me to push. Having dislodged more turds than children in my time, I was fairly convinced of my authority on the subject matter – but they were having none of it. While trying to hold the previous night's badly planned sausage and bean casserole inside, more and more doctors and midwives arrived. Hushed conversations were happening in corners of the room and a horrible sense of déjà vu washed over me. This time, though, I got to the pushing stage and Steve was telling me to keep going, and to try harder ... Lads, if you're reading this – see the previous note about your pie holes when it comes to opinions on our holes. It won't bode well for you. There was also a terrifying female doctor shouting at me from in between my own legs – who did she think she was talking to?!

'I'm not the bloody one you should be shouting at, love! Get down there and tell it to come to your voice!' Felt a bit bad for her in the end, because she did inspire me to deliver something ... but it was full of pork and bean goodness. 'TOLD YOU I JUST NEEDED A POO!'

After that little unplanned delivery, the need to push dissipated, and the anxiety of the room increased tenfold – no one knew how to open the windows. With my legs akimbo, and more and more people arriving (potentially even a passing school trip that had confused the noises coming out of the room for a petting zoo), things were starting to get serious ... Both mine and the baby's heart rates were all over the place, and my temperature was sky high. It was all going tits up and they needed to get the baby out stat. After all the anxiety, pain, and hard work, another emergency section loomed. Instinct had completely taken over – I'd mentally checked out and willingly handed myself over to the professionals. Just as long as they saved her, I didn't care how it happened. Fortunately, they were able to give me a spinal, and my biggest fear of being knocked out again didn't come to fruition. Steve got to stay, and minutes later, from beyond the blue sheet, our little lion queen Evelyn appeared. A girl. My mind was blown. She was placed on my chest to be cradled with my very wobbly Mr Tickle arms – shaking with anaesthetic and shock, I was absolutely terrified of dropping her flat on her beautiful (but somewhat cone-shaped) head. A sobbing Steve went with her as she was whisked away to be checked over by the medical team, leaving me on the table to be put back together. There'd been a fairly big blood loss – apparently a risk of a late-stage C-section – and the doctors were also making comments about a foul smell coming from inside me. 'Errr thanks guys, I'm right here ...' It transpired to be an infection in my womb, the explanation as to why, once again, things hadn't gone to plan. Stitched back together and in recovery, our little circle of life was reunited and we were officially a family of four.

I felt as though we'd had a fairly close call, and funnily enough the same levels of post-section guilt I'd suffered after Jack weren't present. After years of beating myself up about having not done things 'properly', I was at peace with how my daughter entered the world. She was my much-needed wake-up call. If my babies had been birthed as 'nature' had intended, none of us would be here to tell the tale. We survived, and that's the most important thing. Ladies who are about to have Caesareans, ladies who've had them – DO NOT DO YOURSELF A DISSERVICE. C-sections are not the easy way out. Take all the help you are offered, cry as much as you want, but, more importantly, give yourselves the credit you deserve. Women, although we may all be roughly designed the same – there are physiological differences that impact on childbirth massively. My body wasn't built to push people out, especially big ones. My preference for hunky, strapping blokes with broad shoulders (Steve, you're welcome), combined with my narrow pelvis, back in the olden days would have resulted in a death sentence. So why should I feel guilty about being alive? It's proper daft. We're too hard on ourselves … natural, Caesarean, surrogate, adopted … kids don't care how they entered the world – they just care about love, happiness, and snacks … all the snacks.

When it comes to giving advice on being in labour … I don't really have any, other than ditching the birth plan! Go with an open mind (an open cervix helps too) and an ability to go with the flow. I still wonder whether if there hadn't been so much expectation surrounding the moment of Jack's delivery, would there have been as many residual feelings of failure and inadequacy? People are unpredictable, especially little ones, and things can change at the drop of a hat – holding yourself to a prescriptive strategy on how things should happen isn't always feasible and you'll only be left feeling disappointed that things didn't turn out how you'd hoped. It's shit-scary; it's the great unknown – a pivotal moment in your life that changes EVERYTHING. There's no way of knowing how you'll cope in the situation until you've been in it. Also, don't listen to too many people either – birth is like a beautiful, bloody, snowflake … completely individual. What happened to one person more than likely won't happen to you. Just because I had bad labours, it doesn't mean you will; just because your friends are planning on hypnobirthing, it doesn't mean you have to. Just because you're offered all the drugs, it doesn't mean you *have* to take them … but it probably will be the only legal time you'll find yourself in that position. *Carpe diem* and all that …

On the subject of advice, though, I do have a few tips for non-participating partners.

1. Faint: Don't, it's annoying.
2. Panic: Don't, it's annoying.
3. Breathe: Don't, it's annoying.
4. Touch: Don't, it's annoying.
5. Jokes: Don't, it's annoying.
6. Photographs: Don't, it's annoying.
7. Sleep: Don't, it's annoying.
8. Eat: Don't, it's annoying.
9. Leave: Don't, it's annoying.
10. Ask 'what's that smell?': Don't, it's probably a poo.

And for those concerned they too will be struck down with babynesia in the near future, I've taken the liberty of writing a nice little open letter to remind myself not to be so easily swayed …

Dear future me,
Step away from that potato baby.

You already have two children. One of each – healthy and happy. Quit while you're ahead.

You will not, however, remember how much those two 'blessings' physically pained you as they entered the world. You are blinded by your love for them, even though one has probably just curled one out on your living room carpet and the other is licking the dog.

Go look in the mirror at what used to be your belly button – can't see it? That's because it's now under a fold of skin. Lift that up … there you go. Now assess your C-section scar – they've ruined your chances of making it as a Victoria's Secret model …

If you're feeling broody, take yourself back in time, to a dark place when your midwife told you that if you didn't crap yourself while giving birth then you weren't trying hard enough. Do you really want to go back there? No, didn't think so. Go to the toilet in private (well with small children and a dog watching) and relish how nice it is.

Labour can be a beautiful, magical experience for some people. You are not one of them. You birth hulk babies, badly, who enjoy taking the non-conventional routes in all aspects of their lives. Take the hint. Your children are like daft cats that manage to squeeze themselves into tight spaces, but aren't great at getting themselves out. Remember this.

You're years down the line now and you won't be able to remember the exactness of labour pain, just that it hurt a bit. This is a LIE. If you've stubbed your toe recently, imagine the pain 100 times over and in the direction of your cervix.

Dignity. You have a teeny, tiny bit of this back now; any more children and you'll lose it for good. You are also vile in labour. Your only method of communication appears to be via the medium of obscenities, combined with a series of cold and terrifying Morse code blinks. Midwives are hard-working, good people. You were not nice to them.

All too soon you won't remember the pain, the emergency sections, blood loss, complications and infections. You'll be so in love with your little family that you'll want to keep making little versions of you and hubs until either your bank account or womb collapses. The emotions for those little people are unrivalled, but remember … YOU SLEEP NOW! You are able to leave the house without looking like you're being evicted, with 20 bags of belongings and enough bread sticks to make a full-sized replica Eiffel Tower.

There will be pangs of sadness knowing that Evelyn is going to be your last baby. After her, there'll be no more first smiles, laughs or drunken steps (until their actual first drunken steps). The only chubby thighs remaining will be your own. That will suck. As will having to go through all of their teeny tiny clothes and giving away what's no longer required … 100 shit-stained vests you've been holding onto, just in case they're needed again …

Come to think of it … childbirth really wasn't that painful. Yes, it nipped a bit around the edges and there were some physical and emotional scars, but it wasn't that bad – was it? Maybe just the one more …?

8

The After Birth

After months of water-retained, knee-knocking labour fear, you've had a baby. Congratulations! You're now in a super-special club of women who know … antenatal classes are an absolute crock of shit. Not helpful in the slightest. Take your knitted cervix Jane, and shove it up your faff …

Months in the making, sometimes days in the removing – look at what you did! You created a beautiful little human … who looks like a cross between your father-in-law and a pug, and is covered in that white stuff that comes out of bacon when you fry it. With the arrival of new life comes your first taste of the purest, deepest and most unconditional love that any human can experience … for the midwife inserting the pain-relieving suppository. Just take it. Feels weird to begin with but trust me, ease into it and feel the sweet, sweet relief. High on life, love, and bum drugs, the swell of emotion you feel for your newborn baby is completely unrivalled. Showering him or her in a million kisses, it's the only time you'll ever happily put your mouth on anything that's done a stint inside your vagina. So what happens next? Permanent residency on cloud nine? You ride off into the sunset with your ISOFIX sensor beeping the whole way, because you have no idea how to fit the car seat? Well, yes, but not initially, because there's a spot of admin to get through first ... The 'After Birth', and I don't mean placenta.

The After Birth is the highly emotional and incredibly undignified 'WHAT THE ACTUAL FUCK' timeframe after you've delivered your baby. Battered, bruised, traumatised, and with no prior experience of handling your pug-in-law, you're thrown into a completely new world you're in no way, shape, or form equipped to deal with. Absolutely knackered, even if you've had a quick labour, you're physically and mentally drained, and potentially still off your tits too, so what's the next logical step here, people? Probably a decent twelve-hour snooze, right? Sleep it off, wake up feeling refreshed and on your parenting A game? WRONG. You're the proud owner of a human surround-sound speaker who, given the circumstances of how they entered the world, seems pretty unreasonably furious at you. Oh sorry ... somebody pushed so hard to get you out of their body, that *somebody's* bowel dislodged every piece of red meat consumed since the age of twenty. You're welcome.

Good job your partner's there to lend a hand ... Wait, what's that? They're not allowed to stay overnight with you in hospital? HAVE I NOT DONE ENOUGH?! Apparently not. It's 9 p.m. and a stern-looking midwife has rung a bell. Out they go. Post-Jack, the shell-shock was unreal. He was born at 4 p.m., and having spent a few hours coming round from the anaesthetic, by the time we'd been wheeled to the maternity ward there was only enough time for Steve to give us a kiss goodbye before he was turfed out and on his way for Chinese food. My main takeaway, on the other hand, was that after finally discovering what meconium was, I'd never enjoy Marmite ever again. We were totally alone behind our flimsy hospital curtain, and I was unable to move the lower part of my body, or even turn to pick up WrestleMania's 'under six-hours-old' newly crowned champ, without experiencing searing pain. Not wanting to cause a fuss, or keep ringing my buzzer for help every ten minutes, I struggled on, silently sobbing while trying to manoeuvre a resisting member of the opposite sex onto my boobs. Looking back on this with clearer and slightly less traumatised eyes, how bloody foolish. I'd been awake for forty hours, cut open, and still drowsy from all the drugs – if it was heavy machinery being operated instead of a heavy baby, it wouldn't be allowed. I was a learner parent, massively under the influence – someone really needed to take away my keys and get me a fucking Uber. If anyone reading this is about to give birth (sorry about the previous chapter … and well, everything that's about to follow in this one), let me give you some very important words of advice. Asking for help doesn't make you a failure. So please, if you find yourself in a situation where you are struggling, promise me you'll slam your hand down on that buzzer faster than a furious Simon Cowell on *Britain's Got Talent* watching a tone-deaf person take on a Mariah Carey song. PROMISE?

I didn't know what my kid wanted from me … blood? Probably, and from the cord – 'Oi, where did that big straw go?' It would have made life easier for him, because he and I were not exactly at one with breastfeeding from the word go. Did anyone else get shown a video at their antenatal class of a newborn baby, eyes squinting from the brightness of life outside the womb, crawling up its mother's stomach and effortlessly latching straight on to her nips? Yeah … that didn't happen for me – retrospectively a blessing because it resembled a furless mole motor-boating a semi-conscious and half-naked woman. TERRIFYING. No, as initially feared, both my children inherited my ridiculously poor sense of direction, so instead of heading to my gigantic nipples, they furiously tried to suck nutrients out of my stinky, unshaven, post-labour armpits.

With Jack, in the end, his outraged cries must have been doing everyone's heads in so much that a midwife appeared through my curtains, wellies on and pail in hand, ready to hand-milk me. Oh, the indignity … all for about three drops of thick, yellowy, curdled milk, which he gulped out of a syringe then promptly went back to sleep. FOR ALL OF FIVE MINUTES. The lad was nearly the same size as a frozen Christmas turkey, so of course he looked at his vanilla shake and wondered where the hell his Big Mac and fries were.

I'd never really understood how sleep deprivation works as a form of torture, until attempting to sleep on a maternity ward filled with screaming babies. It very much felt as though all us mums had been captured by enemy forces and put there together in a bid to break us so we'd spill government secrets. Tell you what, I was willing to admit *anything* if it meant a peaceful night in my own bed.

One of the few benefits of being permanently awake, especially in the dead of night, is that you get lots of time to inspect your handiwork. It's MAD seeing an actual human being you made; to think they've gone from a microscopic sperm and an egg to a real-life person is absolutely mind-blowing. How easily they could have been another monthly period, or wiped into a crusty sports sock at the side of the bed … Instead, they have a perfect little face you hope will only see love, tiny hairy ears (or is that just my werewolf children?) you pray will only hear kind words, and edible toes ripe for the munching. Their innocence, deliciousness and fragility rocks you to the core. Just like that, you have responsibilities and a life other than your own to protect – they are your whole world, and you are theirs … until they start screaming again, that is, and you can find someone else to fob them off onto. In my case, my personal milkmaid, who again appeared through the curtain but instead of attempting second base, asked whether she should try and syringe feed him some formula instead. FORMULA? What would the 'breast is best' brigade say? Having completely lost control of my left eye from tiredness, and with love bites in my armpits, I really didn't bloody care and gladly took the offer of help and maybe even the opportunity for a snooze. Of course, I didn't sleep a wink. Just lay there wide awake, panicking she was a fake midwife who'd stolen my baby. Turns out she was legit, and returned him half an hour later so he could continue his screeching plight – roping in all the other babies on the ward too for a dawn chorus of high-pitched, ear-piercing hangry screams.

'How's your loss?' Not a question about what your postpartum scales are saying, because you're going to look as though you've still got a child inside you for the immediate future. THIS IS NORMAL. Embrace it, eat some Dairy Milk, and if anyone mentions the words 'bounce back' in your presence, bounce a bag of Doritos off their foreheads. No, this is about blood loss. Now, I was either too busy setting up post-birth drinks at my NCT class and completely missed this, or the topic casually wasn't discussed at any great length, because there was zero preparation in my mind for the extent of bleeding. True story – standing up for the first time after delivery, 40 per cent of my insides fell out onto the floor. Naturally, took that all in my stride … 'STEVE CALL AN AMBULANCE, I'M HAEMORRHAGING!' Luckily, he was very calm in his response. 'Babe, we're already in a hospital, let's ask this medical professional standing next to us with a mop …'

Turns out, it's also perfectly normal. Because of the Caesarean, I'd naively presumed that while they were in there rummaging about for their lost watch, they'd do a complete five-star 'vag'let and clean everything out for me – maybe hang a little heart-shaped air freshener from my flaps. No, they do not do that. They do, however, give you a really lovely, arse-munching, puppy training pad to sit on so you don't mess up their sheets. They made particularly enjoyable rustling noises while I was conversing with my father-in-law.

'What's that noise? Oh, something to catch all my juices – mind my catheter bag when you stand up!'

The sheer amount was *horrifying* – and similar to being in a slasher/adult nappy fetish movie. One of the midwives asked me 'Are you passing 50p clots dear?' What, like a pub fruit machine? Also, nobody said a word about those gigantic Great Wall of China sanitary towels you have to straddle every time you step inside equally large post-birth granny pants. While helping me into them, I'm positive Steve did not at all feel like he'd won the cash jackpot.

Something else that absolutely threw me was how quickly you get turfed out of bed after a human comes out of you, especially after a C-section. As a kid, I had stomach surgery and stayed horizontal for days afterwards, so imagine the surprise when my catheter was out faster than a mum who's got childcare.

'Come on, love, time to go for a shower!'

A jug was thrust into my hand to catch the wee, and up I was hoisted. Honestly, I've had longer periods of recuperation after hangovers – when it wasn't always a person coming out of me, mainly bad life choices, and tequila. Also, why are they so fixated on personal hygiene when for the first two years of parenting you'll never have the time to wash? Projects false hope, that does. Let us stew in our own filth and hair grease so we can acclimatise. Regardless, less than eighteen hours after giving birth, off I zombie-shuffled down the ward. Luckily for Steve, he got to come too. Now, you may have seen some sexy shower scenes in your time but I'm willing to bet they have NOTHING on what went down between me and my husband in that prison-block-esque hospital wet room. Forget *Fifty Shades of Grey*, this was Fifty Shades of … Dismay. Seductively, he thrust me against the slippery off-beige bathroom tiles.

'Take me …' I whispered, clinging to the girth of his strapping shoulders '… to the toilet … and bring the jug.' My heart raced as he used his depleting core strength to drop me, from a great height, onto the accessible loo seat, nearly impaling me on the folding hand rail. He slid his hands between my legs and I let out a low and guttural moan … he'd just bashed my faff with the fucking jug handle. 'I want you …' came my breathy instruction '… to wipe for me – I can't bend properly.' He, however, was too busy rolling my blood-stained surgical stockings down my unshaven legs, his body quivering uncontrollably as he discarded them into a medical waste bin that smelt of meat. Swollen, wet, engorged, and feeling dirty, intense throbbing pulsated through my body. He sensed my urgency and didn't hold back, causing me to gasp as he shot his liquid load all over my face …

'Steve! IT'S IN MY EYES!'

Turns out his only experience of shampooing anyone with hair longer than his own was with the dog. Absolutely diabolical scenes. But worse was to follow. Whether you've had a vaginal birth or a sunroof special, the post-birth poo terror is real. What might happen below the belly button if you overly exert yourself again? What else will fall out? Organs? Another child? After both labours, I'd been given iron tablets because of blood loss, so essentially my fear was that Thor's hammer was going to drop out of my arse. I don't know why hospitals are so insistent on you having a wee before being allowed home, but care not about the boulder of compressed white toast that's about to rip you a fourth hole on the way out. Awful. My advice? Little pushes, painkillers, maybe a prayer to the gut gods, and stay away from

Maltesers for a while – you won't be able to look at them in the same way.

If you think pregnancy hormones are an emotional high, wait until the comedown that hits approximately three days after you've delivered. I always thought the baby blues were a myth, but no, if leaking from most of your other orifices wasn't enough – time for your eyes to get in on the action too. Everything is just TOO DAMN MUCH.

Unfortunately for Steve, and anyone within a five-foot radius, baby blues day also happened to coincide with my going home day. And wow … what a sight to behold that was. Firstly, I'd formed an unhealthy attachment to the woman who anally inserted my drugs – saying goodbye to Sandra was difficult, her tender touch would be missed. Secondly, at home, who would hand-milk me in the middle of the night? After the shower incident, there was concern on my part that if Steve were to take on the role, the end of our marriage might be nigh. Things were also about to become very real … the minute we set foot out of the safety bubble of hospital life we'd have to stand on our own as fully fledged parents, and that was a terrifying prospect. The sobbing started the minute we attempted to put Jack's little snowsuit on. 'STEVE, WHY DON'T HIS ARMS BEND?' Tears cascaded down my face as we headed for the exit, mainly because I was still walking like a member of the undead, but also because my baby (minus a snowsuit) was about to get his first glimpse of the real world … sun, sky, clouds, trees, birds … people hooked up to IV lines having a fag. What if smoke got into his lungs or he developed passive smoking? Within thirty seconds of arriving at the car, the type of parent I was going to be had already been well established – completely neurotic and with the catchphrase 'Don't do that, you'll die!'

With Evelyn, things were just as emotional on day three, but we were yet to make it outside the safety of the hospital walls.

You may recall from the previous chapter the weird smell radiating from my body that made the surgeons recoil in horror as if they'd found an unflushable log in a Wetherspoons toilet. After forty-eight hours of intravenous antibiotics, and with hopes pinned on a great escape the following morning, she broke out in a rash.

Backstory Alert! On the day his sister was born, and not wanting to be outshone by her arrival, Jack broke out in chickenpox. I'd had the virus as a kid, so the doctors were fairly certain she'd be fine, but because of the 'possibility' they had to err on the side of caution. When her bloods came back, there was good news – it wasn't chickenpox. The bad news, however, was that she had raised infection markers and they didn't know why, so she would have to be transferred to the Special Care Baby Unit (SCBU). She was poorly, we couldn't go home, and – even worse – we were going to be separated. I was terrified. Was she going to be OK? What if it was something really serious? You know when you see toddlers cry and they're so hysterical they can't catch a breath? That was me, for a week. Here's where, through these pages, I'd love to reach out and hug the bones off any parent who's had a premature baby, or a poorly baby, and hasn't quite had the straightforward exit from hospital they so desperately desired. We were so incredibly fortunate that, after seven days of antibiotics and monitoring, she was allowed to come home. During our time on the SCBU, we were surrounded by mums and dads who'd been on the most incredible journeys – many having started off in Neonatal Intensive Care Units – and whose first weeks or months of parenting had all taken place inside the stark walls of the hospital. Birds, trees, and sunshine had been replaced with feeding tubes, the beeps of machines, and total uncertainty. For many, their experience was still a long way from being over … despite this, it wasn't a place of sadness but one of strength, light and hope. I had such admiration for the inner reserve of those parents, especially at having to leave their babies every night – something that seemed unimaginable to me. I was only over the corridor in the maternity ward, but the prospect of leaving her was gut-wrenching, especially as I'd started to establish breastfeeding – from my actual boobs this time, not from my pits. Fortunately, the nurses were amazing, coming to get me every time she woke in the night and then allowing me to stay on the ward when I was discharged from the maternity unit and a complete emotional mess at the thought of being estranged from my baby. Believe me when I say I've NEVER been so bloody appreciative of someone's kindness in my entire life.

Seriously, no one *really* tells you about the days that follow giving birth in any great depth – and for sure it's one of the strangest parts. There's so much going on mentally, hormonally, physically – and on top of all that, you're suddenly landed with this little person who speaks a language you don't understand and the interpreter's nowhere to be seen. Yet it's the act of labour that gets all the attention in books, films, and antenatal classes. The postnatal blood, gore and shits are casually left out of the conversation, but don't you think that's the kind of stuff we need to know about? If nothing else, so people can make an informed decision on whether they actually want to put themselves through the process of birthing a child/sausage casserole.

The whole experience is overwhelmingly overwhelming; you're doing something completely new and you're terrified – and do you know what? That's absolutely fine! Your body has changed, things aren't the same ... some bits are squishier, some bits are harder, and your boobs are likely to be as veiny as a weightlifter's biceps. You'll feel like you can't do it, that you're not ready to be responsible for a life – for this teeny tiny person, whose heart wholly belongs to you but beats completely independently. It's the scariest thing in the world knowing they don't come with a charger and a three-point plug. Before having kids, I remember thinking I'd be too scared to ever go to sleep – that I'd have to sit up and watch them all night. Yeah, you get over that … quickly. You'll be so bloody knackered you'll trade your soul for a ten-minute kip sat on a hospital toilet trying to piss into a jug. A very wise person once said to me that when you have a baby, you leave your dignity at the door and pick it up again on the way back out. Honestly, as a birther of two … let me tell you, never has a truer word been spoken.

In the days, weeks and months after you've given birth, all those people in your life who didn't tell you about what you could expect after you've expected will of course be on hand to share their literal 'tit' bits of advice too. 'Have you tried holding them in the rugby position?' 'Have you thought about using a nipple shield?' A shield? Who's going to be shooting at them? You may not feel like much of a superhero for what you've been through, but you are, undeniably, Wonder Woman. Yes, you might be crying at literally everything – 'Look, Steve, that pigeon only has one toe!' And even though you won't feel like it at the time, I can guarantee you this – you will be the best, most robust, hardest, yet softest version of yourself imaginable. If you can get through birth, crawling out of bed with stitches in unimaginable places, repeatedly pulling a puppy training pad out of your arse in front of visitors, and at 4.30 a.m. scraping black tarry poo out of the folds of your child's private parts (all while bleeding heavily from your own), you can get through anything.

9

Mummy

You have a human! It's beautiful, it's magical ... it's producing yellow poo that smells like melted butter. Is that normal? Congratulations, you are now a fully fledged and accountable parent to a completely defenceless life form that relies on you for everything. In a nutshell, it is some serious and next-level Tamagotchi shit. This venture into maturity will be one of joy, frustration, and at times isolation. One thing to remember at the start of this exciting and mind-boggling journey into the unknown is that at no point can you ever throw them in a drawer.

All those months of waiting, wondering, and worrying are finally over – the time has come to finally put theory into practice and go it alone in the big bad world of parenting. Buckle yourselves in, because the first eighteen months of the journey are WILD ... the love, the joy, the bone-aching and delirious tiredness of it all. You might not have passed any legally required competency tests before sitting in the driving seat, but those L-plates are coming off and you, my friend, will be hurtling down the road of highly challenging responsibility at 100 mph for the next 18 years.'

Visitors

In the weeks after bringing home your first bundle of joy, you're a bona fide celeb. Oh, the people can't get enough of you! They're sending flowers, showering you with praise, and rolling out the red carpet – it was white, but postpartum bleeding and all. It's all very lovely, but also horribly overwhelming. By your sixth visitor of the morning, you just want them to leave their M&S Babygro by the front door and fuck off so you can sit with your bits or tits out and cry. Post-section, I was trying to keep myself together, literally holding on to my wound, while manically cleaning my house for the onslaught of cooing guests who were only there to get their hit of new-baby smell. Retrospectively, that smell is vagina. Think about it.

Steve and I barely had time to feed ourselves, taking it in turns to shovel dinner down our faces while the other one rocked or was on milk duty, but yet there we were, preparing charcuterie boards and cream cakes for those coming to sniff what my insides smelt like. By the end of the second week, and on realising most babies' motto is 'sleeping is cheating', we could keep up the pretence no more. The house was an utter shit tip, I looked like a kidnap victim who'd been found in a shed six months later, and the only sustenance being offered to visitors was a stale Tesco Value digestive. Don't get me wrong, it's not that you're annoyed with people's kindness, but sometimes … you just need a minute in private to wallow in your own tears and juices. Now, the exception to high-traffic intrusion is if the child you've brought home is … a sibling. Literally, no one gives a shit. I swear people hadn't even noticed I was pregnant a second time, they'd just presumed I'd stacked on the weight. In our case, it looked a lot like the last one, but with less of the novelty value, and the new-baby smell was completely overwhelmed by the stench of a potty-training toddler doing a crap in a shoe. One of our neighbours actually just shoved a Primark babygrow through the letter box so she didn't have to come in and make polite chit-chat about 'Jack's sister'.

'I don't need to see her, love – I can hear her through the walls.'

Feeding

Brace your babalons, I'm going there … breastfeeding. If I wrote about this topic online, there would be a fierce battle to the death between the 'fed is best' and 'breast is best' brigades. It's funny, isn't it, that the matter of how a woman chooses to feed her *own* child should be a catalyst for so much anger, judgement, and vocal criticism? Not every child takes to breastfeeding, not every woman wants to, and not every woman can. Should anyone be made to feel like less of a mother because of the way they provide nutrients to their baby? Abso-bloody-lutely not. I'm going tell you my experience of feeding my children with no agenda, no superiority and no judgment – simply because it's part of my journey, and at no other point in this book would a line about my husband doing a shot glass of boob milk feel right. Putting my hands up here, breastfeeding was something I was a little apprehensive of – as so very many women are. Was it going to hurt? How would it feel to be classified as a food group? And would my milkshake bring all the boys to the yard? As uncertain as I was of becoming some kind of dairy vending machine, it was something I wanted to try.

After having Jack, in those awful three post-C-section days in hospital, I still hadn't really got the hang of things. Various 'bosom buddies' had visited, showing me different ways of holding him or hand-milking myself, but it didn't ever really feel as though we were a good fit – less like a jigsaw and more opposing ends of magnets, as my boob would go one way and he'd swerve me faster than a one-night stand you bump into at the sexual health clinic the following morning. The latch never felt right, and I was convinced he wasn't getting enough of that good Jersey gold-top milk – was it also meant to hurt so much? Every time he angrily clamped his furious little chops around my engorged nips, it was as if a starved piranha was on the end of them. They were so sore I began to dread the sound of his hungry cries, because I knew what was coming next. I'd never really understood the expression 'toe-curling pain' until living through those early days of breastfeeding, but that's exactly what I experienced with every latch. The day after I came home from hospital, I remember the midwife coming to do her first visit and there I was lying on the bed, starkers from the waist up, desperately trying to stick a baby to my bosom like Velcro. In that moment I realised I'd forgotten to pick my dignity up at the hospital door, and in all reality I probably wouldn't be back for it any time soon.

The following day, things took a turn for the worse with both of us being admitted back into hospital within hours of each other. Jack having had a suspected seizure, and me with potential sepsis. With his wife and son at different ends of the hospital, poor Steve didn't know where to run first. It was such an awful experience and, even though I was legit unwell, the internal failings I felt as a mother who was unable to be with her baby as he was subjected to a spinal tap, an MRI, numerous other tests, and was hooked up to IVs, was horrendous. My first introduction to mum guilt was undeniably one I'll never forget. So why am I telling you this here, while talking about breastfeeding? Well, as it transpired, I actually had a run-of-the-mill chest infection, much less dramatic and makes for a far less exciting story. My body, however, absolutely exhausted from a traumatic labour and trying to mend itself from the C-section surgery, had prioritised battling the infection over producing milk. When Jack's test results came back, they all pointed towards dehydration causing his episode – he hadn't been getting enough fluid from me. It was all my fault … my inadequate supply had starved my baby and put him in actual danger. I was absolutely inconsolable.

With my milk still yet to come in properly, the next few days he was formula fed and chugged it down like a university rugby player downing pints. In that moment I wasn't at all precious about where his nutrition was coming from, and if anyone had dared use the expression 'breast is best' in my presence, I'd have bitch-slapped them with one of my Great Wall of China sanitary towels. He was better and thriving, and that's literally all that mattered. Once the emotion had subsided a little, and the milk flow had increased, there was a bit of me that wanted to try again. Was it guilt? Was it societal pressure? I'm not sure, but what was very apparent was my complete distrust in my body – I'd lost all confidence in relinquishing full control of the feeding responsibilities. Anyway, would he even want to go back for another round on the bitty buffet after the euphoria of hitting the bottle? After all, he didn't choose the chug life, the chug life chose him. To be honest, formula kind of seemed like an easier option all round. Steve could get in on the night feeds and I could see how much he was having, which would help to settle my now completely off-the-scale new-mum anxiety. In the end, mainly to keep my nerves in check, I opted to combination feed him, subbing out a night feed for a bottle for the rest of our milky journey together. I didn't even know it was a thing, and it definitely wasn't an option explored during antenatal classes – or even on any of the mum forums I'd visited. As it turned out, it was the perfect option for us.

I'd love to say I wholeheartedly enjoyed my forays into breast-feeding, rocky start aside, but truth be told … I found it really difficult. The only one in my friendship circle to have a baby, I didn't really have a point of reference or close network to share my experiences with – my child-free and carefree inner sanctum of friends would have thrown up Prosecco all over their non-slipper-clad feet if I'd told them my bleeding nipples were turning the kid's milkshake from vanilla into strawberry. Rock-hard knockers, saturated breast pads, constantly smelling of sour milk, springing leaks on hearing any baby in a five-mile radius cry, and waking up in a completely different type of wet patch than you might have nine months previous … There's so much to take on physically and mentally, especially when you're sleep deprived and living in a constantly heightened emotional state – it can become all-consuming. Yes, Titsville sometimes feels like a lonely place to live. That said, pinned on the sofa, unable to move and five feet away from the remote or your phone, feeds can also be blissful and beautiful bonding moments between you and your baby. It's a time to reflect, feel grateful, and of course demolish a family-sized bar of chocolate – you can eat an extra 500 (healthy) calories a day (Fruit & Nut counts as two of your five a day, right?)

From the comfort of my own home I'd look down at his happy little face when he'd fallen asleep after a good suck (just like his dad), his little clammy cheesy hand entwined around my hair, and think 'bloody hell, I made that'. It was very lovely … and VERY different to our public feeding experiences, which weren't quite as serene, with his wiggly, still fairly resistant nature, and his penchant for punching me in the tits. His windmilling limbs and compete refusal to stop and ask for directions to the dinner-plate-sized nipples meant I'd look more at home topless sunbathing in the Costa del Sol than discreetly breastfeeding in the Costa del Coffee. I'd stupidly get really jealous of seeing other mums confidently whacking a boob out in cafes, parks and supermarkets, but for me the mere thought of it would send me into hot sweats, so I would plan whole days around the boob schedule. If I didn't have a baby hanging off my rack, I'd have a breast pump constantly on the go – mooing away as it drained all the hydration out of my body. Also, nothing beats post-pumped nipples – put Steve off strawberry laces for years. Expressed milk was a lifeline, though, for that one time I went out with my friends and hyperventilated the whole time because I'd left Jack behind. I did find myself falling into that ridiculous trap of feeling like I had to tell everyone it was expressed milk, so as not to get the head-tilt of judgment from other new mums. Honestly, as a new parent you're made to feel as if there's no worse white powder to be caught with than a couple of lines of formula.

Proving that – along with pregnancies and babies – no two breastfeeding journeys are alike, when Evelyn arrived on the scene it was a completely different boob game. Knowing the teet'ing difficulties I'd had with Jack, I was steeled and ready to combination-feed her. As it happens, she took to it like a duck to milky water. In all honestly, with a toddler running around, it was actually quicker and easier to whack her on a boob than it was to sterilise all the equipment and knock up a bottle. It's all circumstance, though – some women find it a breeze, others don't, same for our lovely little babies. I look at my kids now and compare them to their classmates and friends – there's no difference in the ones who were breastfed and the ones who weren't. Yes, scientifically speaking, breast milk may be better for them – I see that and appreciate it. But I also look at what happened to my beautiful little boy and can't help but wonder what would have happened if I hadn't been so hell-bent on feeding him 'myself'. The most important thing is that whatever your decision on breast vs bottle, it's your own. Are you breastfeeding because you want to, or are you doing it because you feel like you have to? If something isn't working for either of you then change it – don't struggle on, feeling the need to adhere to the pressure of society (or worse, the NCT group). Personally, I'm glad I gave it another shot with Jack, and then Evelyn – I'd wholeheartedly encourage anyone who's had a challenging experience first time round not to be disheartened in the future. If you also want to press a button and whip up a bottle faster that you could knock up a caramel macchiato – then you do you.

Sleeping

Nothing prepares you for the sleep deprivation. All that third-trimester crap about the reason you can't sleep being because it's your body's way of preparing for what's to come – lies. Tell you what would be more indicative of the truth – the SAS selection process. Ten minutes' sleep and off up the Brecon Beacons you go – and when you get back down, any chance you could spend the day making funny faces, changing nappies every twenty minutes, and pretending to the health visitor you are totally fine?

For a solid month Evelyn woke every hour on the hour for feeds. As I was breastfeeding her, there was nothing anyone else could do to help me. It was a form of torture. My head was constantly foggy, and throbbed from the deprivation of REM – it felt like the end of the world as I knew it. I used to lie there in the dead of night, eyes propped open with matchsticks (the mint chocolate variety), terrified of falling asleep while she was still on me, and silently plotting ways to murder my blissfully content and unconscious husband in his slumber. When she cried, that fucker's eyes didn't even twitch. I'd sometimes hold her – angrily screaming with a sonic boom's ability to shatter an eardrum – right next to his lug holes. Nothing. My hypothetical murder weapon of choice was a milk-saturated breast pad to his open, drooling, snoring gob. Of course, I'd never do it … who'd put the bin out? But I thought about it, especially when he'd wake up in the morning, yawn, stretch his arms above his head, and turn to me saying 'She had a good night, didn't she?'

People just love to chip in with their two cents' worth as well, don't they? My favourite is 'sleep when they sleep'. This would be very useful, apart from the fact THEY NEVER FUCKING SLEEP. Also, if you have another child, you can hardly just go for a catnap and leave them alone with a crate of Play-Doh and a pack of Sharpies.

It's when dealing with a bad sleeper that you're likely to have your first encounter with an absolute PRICK – that's a Parent Releasing Inner Competitive Knobiness. A horrific disorder sadly affecting nearly one in three parents globally. Symptoms develop quite soon after childbirth and include a need to one-up fellow mums and dads at all times, often inciting severe cases of rage and inferiority among those they interact with. Lurking in the shadows of baby classes, health-visitor waiting rooms, and even playgrounds, PRICKs are everywhere. Despite knowing your child is yet to sleep through for longer than a minute, they'll be boasting of how their child has been sleeping for that highly elusive twelve hours a night since leaving the womb.

'Have you tried controlled crying?'

'Yes. Actually, I like to lock myself in the toilet and weep for a total of twenty-five minutes. No more, no less. Oh, you meant the baby …'

Personally, I opt for the 'rocking them for three hours while singing fifty choruses of "Twinkle Twinkle Little Star" until they drift off or your spine crumbles' method. The dummy, or pacifier, is another divisive topic. On hearing horror stories about crooked teeth and 30-year-olds refusing to give them up, we debated whether or not to give one to Jack … for all of five minutes. We quickly realised if we shoved it in, the noise temporarily stopped. A no-brainer. I think you can always spot a baby who doesn't sleep well: seven dummies clipped to its body, and dressed head to toe in 'I love Mummy' clothing, its parents trying to convince themselves their child doesn't actually hate them and isn't trying to kill them slowly through extreme tiredness.

Isolation

One of the biggest challenges many new parents will face that's not often spoken about is how isolating it can be. Yes, the love you have for your child is incredible and magical – I still cry myself to sleep some nights thinking how lucky I am. But there's also a sense of disconnect from your old lifestyle and who you once were. My world was suddenly turned completely upside down, and although I was never on my own (thanks to a small child constantly hanging from me), I had never felt lonelier. When Steve went back to work and I had to fly solo, it was terrifying. Off he causally popped in the mornings to talk to other grown-ups, who'd had more than three hours sleep and were wearing matching shoes, without a care in the world. I wasn't bitter at all. You know what they say … absence makes the heart grow passive aggressive.

My biggest obstacle was actually leaving the house. Having 'disorganisation' as one of your main character traits pre-baby does not serve you well once the high-maintenance bun is out of the oven. This was something I learnt the hard way. The sheer number of items required for a two-hour excursion does not lend itself well to a haphazard approach to life. Nappies, wipes, muslins, milk, dummies, thermometers (medical, room, and bath – anything above 19°C and they spontaneously combust), Calpol, mobile sterilisers, and a cuddly toy. Remembering everything was like being on *The De-generation Game*. By the time I'd got everything into the car, ran back for things I'd forgotten, wrestled a starfish of a baby into a highly restrictive seat, put on my own belt and attempted to drive away, there it was … the arse-rippling nappy-noise of doom, followed by the unmistakable scent of buttery Lur-kak. Back in the house and cutting a child out of a completely yellow vest, I'd be texting full-blown LIES to the person I was meant to be meeting. 'On my way, just stuck in traffic!' Truth be told, it'd be at least another half an hour before we'd be setting foot out of the door. Little tip for you here – when faced with a poonami of epic proportions, the vests with envelope openings at the top are so you can roll them down instead of dragging digested curdled milk through your child's eyes and hair. Only discovered that about two years too late.

Finally on my way, I'd be faced with crippling anxiety about whether the baby was OK in the back of the car. What if they were choking on a bit of blanket fluff, or if they were too hot? I'd eventually arrive hours after I was meant to be somewhere, just as everyone else was leaving. Most of the time, the effort involved in leaving the house didn't feel justifiable in comparison to the reward. Baby classes were a prime example of this. Not my bag at all, sitting in a church hall watching your baby lick contaminated musical instruments while forcing a conversation about weaning with a mum much more together than you – all over a shit cup of coffee and a stale biscuit. It was, however, a focal point in the week, something to work towards and try to get to on time. Never happened. I'd look at other women, out and about, seemingly having left the house without any of the same drama I'd experienced, and wonder 'how the bloody hell do you do it?' I thought I was such a failure, an absolutely rubbish mum, inadequate, and that there was no point in trying to do anything or go anywhere. What I didn't realise was that most of those ladies probably also felt the same way too, but were just better at fronting than I was, smiling on the outside, still leaking from the inside. It's all very scary, new, and not at all similar to the life we were once familiar with. It's totally normal to say it's hard, that it's not what you thought it'd be, and that sometimes you don't enjoy parts of it. It does not make you a bad person who doesn't love their child. It makes you a perfectly rational human being who, in contrast to popular social media life-coaching phrases, 'has not got this'. Most of the time, the only thing I felt I'd 'got' was mastitis and a bill for Baby Sensory classes that we only attended a third of. The best thing to do is not compare yourself, or your children, to anyone else. Social media platforms can be wondrous places that have the ability to connect so many like-minded souls – but they can also be minefields of facades and untruths, provoking the demons in your mind that already make you feel like the turd you can constantly smell on yourself but can't work out where it's coming from. My advice to anyone feeling like this is to only follow those who uplift, not drag down.

Milestones

Bloody obsessed, aren't we? People have those cards they like to place around their babies' heads, like the strangest of tarot readings. 'Today, I pissed in Mummy's open mouth!' There is, however, something so utterly wondrous and special about when your child begins to interact with the world – and you – for the first time. Those smiles, cheeky giggles, and the full-on belly laughs are some of the most spectacularly heart-warming moments you'll experience as a parent.

Your baby's developmental stages are, however, where you'll start to encounter the majority of PRICK behaviour. As with sleeping through the night, there comes an obsession with needing to know if a child can do a variety of tricks, like supporting their own heads, pushing themselves up, and rolling over like dogs, which apparently makes them superior and much more likely to excel at world domination, and Crufts. As someone whose kids are constantly on the go, climbing walls and abseiling off light fixtures, I don't know why we're all so keen to get them moving at such an early age. Jack literally refused to do anything until he was twelve months; in fact, he didn't even start crawling until his first birthday. No fool, he knew if he just sat there not doing anything I'd have to pick him up and carry him places. Kid was street smart. Others were, of course, always on hand to make me 3 a.m. panic-Google whether or not his disinclination to move was normal or not. 'Oh is he not even crawling yet? Jessica's been walking since eight months!' Knob off! You can take great joy in knowing that while the parents of those overachieving mini Usain Bolts are legging it around their houses bubble-wrapping sharp edges, you'll be sat on the sofa, hot drink in hand, watching *This Morning* and overseeing your blissfully happy and perfect baby licking biscuit crumbs off the dog's face.

It's also funny how much more relaxed you are about your second child's development. There's no laying of favourite toys just out of reach to try and entice them to crawl. No, while you're cleaning up after an older sibling who's taken to peeing anywhere that's not in a potty or a toilet, they need to stay incarcerated in that baby bouncer for as long as you can get away with. A major takeaway point here is that our babies are only small – and still – bundles of chub once, so let's not wish their little lives away; and secondly, it's a bloody nightmare once they do learn how to move – so just enjoy the calm before the 'running at full pelt into doorframes and coffee tables' storm.

'Isabella just loves a kale, broccoli, and spinach puree!' No, she doesn't, she just has no point of reference or vocal ability to tell you she thinks your ice-cube trays full of unseasoned sludge look and taste like swan shit. Yes, the race to a perfectly weaned, organic-carrot-stick-eating baby is THE one to win. I challenge you to go into any coffee shop on a weekday morning and not find a bunch of mums trying to outdo one another with NutriBullet recipes.

'Annabel Karmel said to use sweet potatoes, but I think it tastes so much better with rutabaga!' Cue lots of agreeing and nodding, followed by sloping off to the toilet to google 'what the fuck's a rutabaga'.

'We're so lucky – she eats everything we put in front of her!'

So does your baby – very partial to tablemats, coasters, small chokeable pieces of Lego. You smile, nod, then feed your own child yet another bag of rice cakes. Weaning is a big milestone, one that transforms your babies from milk-guzzling little beauties into real-life human beings who require utensils and cups to throw across the kitchen. You'll have a camera roll filled with 19,863 photos of them smiling with varying shades of crud encrusted over their beaming yet minging faces. When we weaned Jack, two weeks early (don't tell the health visitor as I'm fairly sure it's still an arrestable offence), the poor kid was fed baby rice mixed with formula – effectively milky sawdust. In another classic example of first child vs second, from about eight months Evelyn was on fish fingers and bags of chocolate buttons.

The all-important first word – what will it be? Who will it be? The tension among the antenatal friendship group is palpable. Of course, there's always one type, not mentioning any names, who thinks their child is already fluent in the English language.

'Oh, little Freddy said his first word when he was three months old. Agoo.'

'Is 'agoo' actually a real word?'

'It's actually a place in the Philippines. He's incredibly cultured you know.'

Of course he is. He certainly looks it, licking your bifold window and spreading a Dairylea triangle all over the floor.

When your partner's out of earshot you can't help but prime them for a 'ma-ma' – it's only fair, isn't it? You're mostly the one de-snotting their nostrils with your homemade fingernail chisel. Of course they are going to say your name first … 'Say Ma-ma. MA MAAAAAAAAAAAA.'

'Da-da.'

'What? No! Ma-ma. MA MAAAAAAAAAAAA.'

'Da-da!'

'No, shhhhh!'

'Da-da, Da-da, Da-da, Da-da, sssssssssshhhhhhhhhh!'

For fuck's sake. It's at that precise moment you realise that for months your partner has been doing exactly the same thing behind your back – prepping them at every opportunity to say their name instead of yours. What a pair of PRICKs.

Flying the nest

For many, there comes a time when your baby will need to fly the nest – it'll happen sooner than you think, and you will NOT be ready for it. Nursery. Entrusting the care of your child into the hands of another person is one of the most gut-wrenching things a parent can do. How do you even go about making the right decision on where they should go? Who is worthy of such a sacred task? In our case, we just picked the one that smelt the best. Job done.

My biggest wobble was the night before, seeing Jack's little bag packed and ready to go by the front door … as though he was off to the office in the morning and might not be back for dinner. I sobbed so much my mascara ran down my face and into my spaghetti bolognese. Was I a bad mother? Maybe I shouldn't have been going back to work … That was it, I was calling work in the morning to quit and I was going to look after him until he was forty-two. Steve had to talk me down from the career-suicide ledge, reminding me it was just his settling-in morning … he'd be gone for an hour and I'd have to sit in reception and wait for him the whole time, watching him eat crayons on a monitor. A valid point. The abandonment guilt was unreal, though. Steve, on the other hand – not arsed. Now, I'm not insinuating he loves his children any less, because of course that's not true. I think it's just that society is still so geared to the MENtality of women staying at home and raising the children while the men plough on at work – we feel the culpability deep within our psyche, and womb. Things are beginning to change for the better, with more efforts being directed at parental leave and equality measures, but I think more needs to be done in terms of shifting our own mindsets too. Our partners are half responsible for that child too, our jobs are equally as important as theirs – so why do we solely burden the guilt that comes with wanting or needing to provide for our families?

My job, at the time, wasn't set up for flexible working in the slightest. When I posed the question of a part-time position it was met with a big fat 'no' because it would, apparently, create a 'precedence'. Heaven forbid that a company employing predominantly women in their twenties and thirties would want to appear considerate towards those choosing a career and a family! It played horribly into the age-old narrative of women not being able 'to have it all'. It's really quite sad it's taken the Covid pandemic for women to prove working from home and flexible hours are practical, productive, and prosperous. In my case, I quit my job – only to be taken back on immediately by my employer as a freelancer. It would seem to be more socially acceptable for a member of the team to be part-time if they were not officially affiliated. The flip side of contract life was that I charged them three times as much, left all responsibility at the door, and gave fewer shits about having to leave at 4 p.m. to do the nursery pick up. The negatives were, of course, no holiday or sick pay, meaning that when a nursery virus swept through the house, I got nothing for having my head down a toilet for a week (apart from more germs).

From poosplosions to non-raving all-nighters, attempting to eat out with a screamy baby to hysterically scrambling round on a barber's floor collecting precious first locks (and beard hair of middle-aged men), the first venture into parenting is daunting, yet truly brilliant. Unexpected bumps in the road will be hit, and the experience might not be exactly what you'd imagined. It's a stomach-churning roller coaster you can never get off, quite often leaving your mental and physical reserves running on empty. EVERY day is a school day … there are mistakes (anyone else ever machine-washed a shitty disposable nappy?); close calls with sharp-edged kitchen units; and plagues of guilt one minute, followed by torrents of joy the next. We're kept constantly on our toes, like coiled springs, ready for danger – emotional and exhausted bodyguards who are protecting the most precious cargo in the world while undertaking unpaid on-the-job training. Something worth stating to anyone who's yet to have a child and is thinking of preparing themselves with dog ownership first: it's not a realistic way of bracing yourself for what's to come – you absolutely can't put them on a lead or tie them to a lamp-post while you pop into the shops, frowned upon … apparently. Also, no matter how difficult life seems after the arrival of your first baby, it's going to be more chaotic, but less neurotic, when the second (third, fourth, fifth, sixth …) comes along. For sure, there are certain things you'll be more relaxed about second time round, like weaning, sleeping, clothes – everything's a hand-me-down when you're second out, including the womb.

When Jack's umbilical cord fell off we kept it, like the way people do with their dehydrated wedding flowers – but more disgusting. Popped it in his baby book so he had something to freak him the fuck out when we're dead and he's cleaning out the loft. With Evelyn, hers fell off and the dog ate it. Again, people – first child vs second child!

Moral of the story, the first couple of years of your child's life is actually only a very short time. It may feel like the difficult times are never ending, and that there'll never be a life beyond the crazy baby-bag lady 'IF YOU'RE TIRED THEN JUST GO THE FUCK TO SLEEP' haze. But during the good times, it terrifyingly goes by in the blink of an eye … suddenly they are running, talking, reading, and you have no idea where that tiny little baby who used to barf in your hair has gone. You'll mourn the loss of all of those stages you once thought to be challenging – take it from a woman who cries every time her husband suggests going through the mountains of baby clothes from four years ago and sending them to the charity shop. 'STOP THROWING AWAY MY MEMORIES!'

Children do everything in their own time (this will become apparent when you ask them to put on their shoes in later life) so try not to compare them, or your own parenting abilities, to others. Also, ask for bloody help! Put out an SOS to friends and family, then treat yourself to a shower, throw on your PJs, and enjoy a warm drink that hasn't been microwaved three times. NO WOMAN IS AN ISLAND. Although some, at times, may wish they were. The Virgin Islands.

Two things in life are certain when you become a parent. The first is that despite promising you'll never do it, you'll be that person who sniffs their child's arse. Fact. No getting away from it. Embrace it – sometimes it's the only way of knowing if it's a nappy change or a phantom poo. The second is that once they've arrived, you cannot imagine what life would be without them … probably quieter, and with a much cleaner house. But potentially not quite as much fun …

10

Vulvarine

Having a baby does a lot of strange things to your body that I was NOT aware of before committing to the process, and, if I'm being honest, I was too busy worrying about a vaginal apocalypse to bother Googling what was going to happen in the years to come. Is she going to be ripped in half like a garlic tear-and-share loaf? Is someone going to come at her with a knife, and a crochet needle? And will things be so bad 'down there' you'll make your partner sign a DNR (DO NOT REPRODUCE) order? After giving birth, there are actually far more pressing matters at hand than your vag, because believe me when I say that no one's going to be looking at it for a while – yourself included.

It's the sneaky, lesser-known changes you need to worry about – ones the Illumumnati, a secret society shrouded in mystery and incontinence pads, have kept hidden from all women of child-bearing age for centuries, presumably in a bid to keep the human race alive. Only when talking to fellow members of this secret sect does it become apparent you are not an anomaly in the system ... these are common ailments, and the deceit feels OUTRAGEOUS. How could you have got so far into the process without somebody pulling you to one side and telling you trampolines and groin sweat will be your arch nemesis? It's criminal, there should be a tribunal. But whatever curveballs (otherwise known as piles) your post-baby body throws at you, let me offer some reassurance in the fact you're most definitely not alone ...

Seriously, what happens to our bodies is the stuff of actual nightmares. My friend Claire (name changed so as not to be sued) is now too embarrassed to attend her son's football matches after celebrating one of his goals a little too enthusiastically. The cacophony of wind released from her arse rerouted itself up through her flaps, and boomed around the pitch like a chorus of *vulva*zelas going off at the World Cup. Forget lecturing teenagers on the dangers of unwanted pregnancies and sexually transmitted diseases – just show them a picture of a postpartum nipple with a six-inch black hair hanging out and they'll be begging for the condoms.

To set the scene, here's a picture my then five-year-old drew, proudly exclaiming, 'Mummy, it's you!'

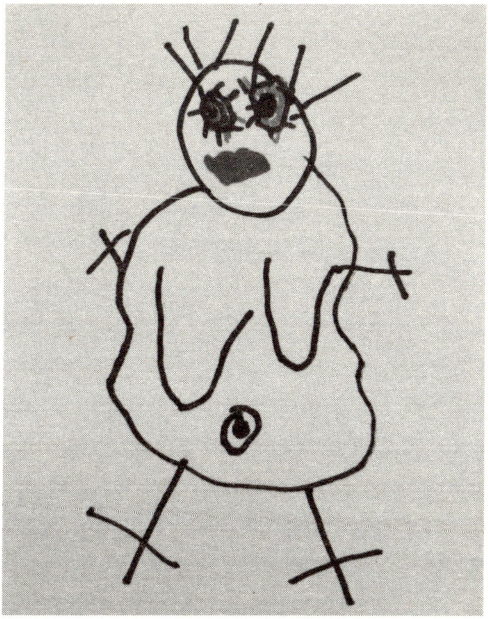

'Awwwww, thank you, sweetheart! Now off you pop to the naughty step ...' Sadly, this atrocious depiction of Jabba the Hut on a night out is a fairly accurate portrayal of postpartum life. The love I hold for my children is unrivalled, when they're behaving, but not only did they destroy my ability to drink more than two glasses of wine without hugging the toilet bowl, they wreaked absolute havoc on my body.

One of my biggest grievances is my hair, something I'm still grappling with five years after my last baby was born. Nature giveth, and nature taketh away ... because when you're pregnant, you're blessed with an amazing head of hair. Don't ask why, but for some evolutionary reason, maybe to make up for labia the size of bratwurst, you get given great pregnancy locks. Very much in the realms of a Crufts show dog, with a gloriously thick and glossy coat, you're lured into a false sense of security as you prance around thinking 'Yaaaaas, because I'm woof it!' And while you're all Afghan Hound up top, downstairs you're living your absolute best life as a weird hairless terrier thanks to a halt in leg-fur and pube production. 'How lovely!' you think. It is, however, one of nature's cruellest tricks, and only discovered eight months after giving birth when you look down in the shower and find more hair in the plug than the pre-holiday bikini shave. Sorry, what now? How did you sit through hours of antenatal classes, looking at curry pastes in nappies, and not one fucker cared to mention you'd be left with a receding hairline best resembling nineteen-eighties Bruce Willis? On top, follicles may have appeared to 'die hard', but downstairs your bush hair is multiplying at the rate of Gremlins, adopting the appearance of Brian May's head stuck in a pair of knickers. In fact, there's so much, you begin to question whether some of it could be transplanted to your scalp because up there you're malting handfuls, and brush-loads, at a time. You're picking it out of your child's food, bedding, nappy, and from around your husband's penis in a newly formed woollen cock ring. Tumbleweeds of the stuff lurk in corners of your house, mating with pet fur to make a hybrid of super-allergies. Let's face it, your hairline is a total mess. Bald patches, different colours, random wiry pube-esque antennae – we just need to chuck it all up in a ponytail and be done with it. Easier said than done, though, because up-dos are no longer your friend, ironically, along with mum buns. The minute you tie up what's left, you're gifted with two spiked devil horn tufts that defiantly stick up no matter how much Elnett Extra Strong Hold you throw at them. No, nothing can restrain them, they're the Chumbawamba of the hair world – they get knocked down, but the little bastards keep getting back up again. Upsettingly, I'm now faced with the stark realisation my hair might always look as though I've instigated a late night catfight in a kebab shop.

If eyes are the windows to the soul, I worry what that my bloodshot, tired, and barely open pissholes say about my psyche

– they perfectly depict a confused mombie who very rarely knows why she's walked into the same room four times. What is she looking for? Why is she there? And why has she just bumped into the Hoover and apologised to it? Yes, baby brain is very real and not just a pregnancy phenomenon. There were several points after having Jack when my own sanity was called into question, by me. I went from being a woman with a serious (ish) job to forgetting about the same load of washing in the machine six times in the space of three days. What had become of me? Was it normal to cry for a month straight because I couldn't find my slippers? Instigated by pregnancy hormones, and then cemented by months and sometimes years of sleep deprivation, the fog feels unlikely to ever lift … even when it dissipates slightly, you'll probably still be on your hands and knees looking for AWOL footwear – which you will, of course, be wearing.

Only occasionally does a scatty memory work to your advantage – for example, casually forgetting the promise of a birthday blow job. Other times, however, it can leave you terrified you'll never be able to run at full mental capacity again, or that you'll leave a child outside Asda. It's not just a case of being forgetful either – sometimes I'm absolutely convinced there's a direct correlation between me having kids and not possessing the necessary brain cells required to help them with their primary school maths homework. 'Mummy, shall we just ask Google?' Not content with hair, the hormones also stole my clever. Could have been worse, could have pinched my teeth – because that's also a thing. Have a baby, they said. It'll be fun, they said! No one said a jot about going from 'yummy mummy' to 'gummy mummy'. Are unborn vampire foetuses chugging calcium from their mothers as though they're a never-ending McDonald's milkshake? Well, that's what those old wives' tales would have you believing, but it's actually more to do with our good friends the hormones again – changing the pH balance in our mouths.

Who'd have thought it, hey, a pregnant woman with an acidic tongue? Although, I imagine eating a six-pack of Snickers Ice Cream Bars at 3 a.m. also doesn't help cavity matters …

What about skin? Doesn't having a baby make your skin glow? Well, yes, but that's mainly from the exertion of projectile vomiting ginger nuts. If you were expecting to exude the radiance of an ethereal being during your pregnancy but ended up with acne, broken veins, skin tags, chin hairs, and teenage oil slicks – post-baby, things aren't much better. Why did no one tell me about melasma? No, not Donald Trump's wife but a skin condition leaving you with patches of discoloured skin all over your mush. Also known as a 'pregnancy mask', this absolute corker of a dermatological clusterfuck made its first appearance on my mug a few months after Jack was born, choosing to mark its arrival subtly … above my top lip. That is correct, it was like I'd got drunk on a hen party and had a fake moustache tattooed onto my face. Couldn't wax it, couldn't cover it, and if my face went anywhere near the sun, it got ten times darker. For six whole months I had to walk around as the spitting image of Borat. Never mind a pregnancy mask, a surgical mask wouldn't have gone amiss – where was a pandemic when I needed it? Just when the melasma finally seemed to settle down, Evelyn arrived … as did an outline of the African continent on my forehead. It's true what they say about the sun ageing you, because I've now adopted the fashion sense of a factor 50 and visor wearing OAP. To add insult to injury, my face is super sensitive to the sun, but other parts of my body have gone the other way, becoming impervious to sunlight. My shins, for example, no longer tan. NOT AT ALL. Oh, but my thighs and feet do, so on a lovely July day I've got legs that resemble a freshly shaved doner kebab.

And, of course, the post-breastfeeding boobs! Having never really had more than a handful before, I quite enjoyed the arrival of the huge pregnancy hooters, despite their blue veiny appearance. The problem with things becoming overly inflated, as anyone who's ever slept on an airbed will tell you, is that what goes up must come down. Lo and behold, pretty much a month or so after I'd finished breastfeeding, the mosquito-esque hiss of air emitting from my chest was almost audible, as they slowly went from perky to pancakey. It was at this point all the stretch marks I thought I'd escaped during pregnancy reared their ugly heads, same for my stomach too. 'Tiger stripes' my arse; instead, I had hundreds of silvery trails everywhere, as though a bunch of snails had enjoyed an orgy on my baps.

I'd be curious to know how much of an impact breastfeeding had on my boobs VS the toll of pregnancy itself, because I'm highly suspicious a lot of the damage was actually done before Operation Dairy Cattle began. Regardless, what can you do? Bar a boob job, this is what I have now and I'm just going to have to work with the wonky handful that's been dealt. Positivity is key, despite now being a cup size half-empty kind of girl. Can a bowl of cereal be rested on them? No. On lying flat on my back, do they slide off my chest like butter on hot potatoes? Yes. And when on all fours (a rarity), do two perfectly pointy Dairylea triangles droop off my chest and graze the ground beneath me? Absolutely ... but they have served me well over the years, feeding my babies and getting me into many a nightclub before it was technically legal – so for that, I'm eternally grateful to them. Shit happens and boobs drop. Gravity comes for us all at some point or another – no one is safe, not even men. We might be tucking our knockers into our knickers, but ladies, take some solace in knowing they'll be tucking their bollocks into their socks.

My stomach – that's destroyed too. After having kids, much like Britain debating whether it wanted to leave the EU, my bellybutton had no idea whether it was an inny or an outy. Its position now heavily depends on how much bread I've eaten.

Half a French stick and boom! Out it pops, a little belly button boner. Breadxit, if you will. The low carb days aren't much better – when bloating retreats, all that remains is a cat's puckered arse hole, so cavernous it gives the back of the sofa a run for its money. Evelyn once stuck her finger in it and pulled out £7.50! As well as loose change, there's also a lot of loose skin just hanging around, adopting the stretchable capabilities of a Marvel superhero, which is always helpful in case the need for a skin graft arises, or the kids need a windbreaker at the beach.

My belly button, stretchy bits, and snail trails aren't the only midriff casualty of pregnancy, however ... introducing 'diastasis recti'! No, not an eighties synth band but a separation of your abdominal muscles. My very beautiful but larger than average babies certainly left their mark on my stomach, and by mark I mean a vast void in my gut to rival the Grand Canyon. What causes it? And will everyone who gives birth end up with a hole big enough to smuggle litre bottles of gin through customs? Well, it depends on how much your connective tissue has thinned out to accommodate your expanding womb, and whether you're a fairly petite female who has a tendency to grow Hulk babies. Not pointing fingers, but I'm pretty convinced it was Jack's stint on the inside that was responsible for the initial perimeter break – then when Evelyn arrived, she smashed her way through the remaining wall as though it was 1989 Berlin.

Because both of mine exited via the sunroof, I'm also blessed with a little something called the C-section shelf – a marsupial pouch that sits above the Caesarean scar. No matter how much your weight changes, or how many ab crunches you attempt, that bumbag of human flesh ain't going anywhere apart from down south and towards your vagina – leaving you looking like Skippy the bush kangafoo. It's the last line of defence between you and tight-fitting clothing, and can only be defeated, temporarily, by a pair of reinforced control pants akin to an adult wetsuit.

But I think it's time we addressed the elephant (ears) in the room … minnies, muffs, pussies, vajayjays, fannies, front bottoms – whatever the name, she's many women's biggest worry when it comes to arriving at motherhood. During our pregnancies, we all say things along the lines of 'I hope the baby is happy and healthy', and we do, but in our minds we follow that statement up with 'and that my vagina won't be left with the same storage capabilities as a Volvo estate'. Will she still look and feel the same? How about sex? No offence to male partners, and of course their massive willies, but what if it's akin to lobbing a pencil down a corridor? What if, after being stretched so far, our vaginas will have the internal elasticity of tumble-dried tights – baggy AF and constantly down by your ankles? As my two were both delivered 'unnaturally' in theory things down there should have come away relatively unscathed. In theory … Wait, what's that? If you've had a C-section your bits are still screwed?! Well, not in a sexual way … because my body was having absolutely none of that nonsense. Something no one tells you about the early months of motherhood is that hormones continue to wreak havoc on our bodies, and their fluids, for months after giving birth. If you've chosen to breastfeed, you'll find yourself constantly dehydrated, but there's also another more worrying drought happening … in your nether regions. Drier than the Sahara. Yes, soreness, itchiness, burning, and tightness are the key personality traits of your newest, hairiest, sexy-time-fighting sidekick … Vulvarine.

Just as one part of the female anatomy has been reduced to dust, another's suddenly as free-flowing as the Amazon. Enter bladder weakness. Cold season in my house is also more commonly referred to as monsoon season – one sneeze and the kids are reaching for their galoshes. My bladder resents the term 'weak'; she's the Beyoncé, Kelly, and Michelle of the organ world. 'Excuse me, I am strong, I'm independent …' until it comes to shouting too loudly for the TV to be turned down and then 'Destiny's Had a Child' is on her knees, sat in a puddle of her own piss. Yes, pelvic floor exercises probably should have been done during pregnancy, but at the time it just seemed a lot of hard work. In my defence, the sensation of doing them totally weirds me out and – you cannot convince me otherwise of this – I swear that muscle is directly attached to your eyebrows. You're now sat there doing a few cheeky squeezes, aren't you? It's a natural instinct the minute people mention them – same with yawning. What are your eyebrows doing? See! Possibly I should have made more of an effort after Jack was born but because he was a section, there was a huge – and very wrong – presumption they wouldn't need to be done. He hadn't been pushed out, so surely that was a get-out-of-jail-free card? What I'd failed to realise was that before being forcibly removed from my womb, all 10 lb 10 oz of him had jumped around on those pelvic muscles like Kris Kross at a trampoline birthday party. Absolutely destroyed. There is some good news to be had, however, because in a LOT of cases bladder weakness is totally fixable. Sometimes women have a slight tendency to just presume the occasional gush of wee is an acceptable part of postpartum life, or an unavoidable knock-on of getting older, but that really doesn't have to be the case with the right corrective exercises. So come on, all together now … one, two, three, SQUEEZE!

If the above gynaecological issues weren't bad enough, enter player two … the pelvic prolapse. For the record, I'm 'anti' anything that involves organs tumbling out of your body in the fashion of KerPlunk. Imagine being told, pre-enlisting for the job of continuing the human race, there'd be a chance your insides would make a break for the outside – who would have still signed on the dotted line? Not bloody me! At the very least I'd have insisted on seeing the contract and adding a break clause … break me, and I'm fucking out. It does happen, to lots of women – as do the dreaded bum grapes of doom. Ahhh, piles – what a pain in the arse. Nothing quite beats that itchy, stabbing, can't sit down properly feeling! What a way to reward a woman for her services to humanity by gifting her swollen blood vessels that resemble a nice new pair of dangly earrings. Where are the Blue Peter badges, Pride of Britain awards, or MBEs? The good news here is that there are lots dignified ways of treating them, such as an ice pack wrapped in a tea towel, cream from your local pharmacy while half the people in your road are waiting for their prescriptions, rubber band ligation, electrotherapy, and, of course, you could just go ahead and shove them back inside your own arse … or let your partner – who doesn't love kinky times with anal beads?

Of course, the hormonal Russian roulette doesn't just point and shoot at your body. It's coming for your head, too. Pre-babies, I was an emotionally void fortress of calm and rationality. Post-babies, I'm somewhat less stable when it comes to TV charity fundraisers and adverts for donkey sanctuaries. There's also a need to tell my kids I love them fifty times a day otherwise we might all die. Cuckoo, I know. It makes no sense … but death lurks behind every corner when you have kids – non-tepid water, paedophiles, uncut grapes, and people who've smoked in the past ten years. 'DON'T YOU TOUCH MY BABY!' Don't get me started on a unsterilised dummy, either – you'd throw yourself on top of that germ-multiplying grenade to prevent your precious firstborn from putting it anywhere near their gob. 'SOMEBODY BOIL A KETTLE!' Second born, you just flick off the dog hair and shove it back in. Also, I'm quite partial to sneaking into my kids' bedrooms while they're fast asleep, face about an inch away from theirs, and creepily whispering, 'Mummy loves you so much', while ugly-crying. When my husband does the bedtime routine he puts them in their rooms, shuts the door and doesn't see them again until morning. 'See ya, losers!' All while crazy train over here is there with a hand on their backs, checking for the rise and fall … and wielding a digital thermometer in their sleeping faces. God help them if they have a temperature, because it's always worse-case scenario – it's never just a cold or just a rash, it is ALWAYS some kind of terrible tropical fever. Obviously, it's never because I've smothered them in three duvets and it's June.

Ladies, we're all normal … don't panic. If you're worried something weird is going to happen to you, or it is happening right now, I guarantee you that there will be millions of women who've already trod those boards. From smelling of onions, to night sweats and rapidly growing ogre feet, from weird sexy dreams to an expanded ribcage that's given you the wingspan of a pterodactyl – these are the sacrifices we make in the name of motherhood. We have created beautiful human beings, perfect in every way, much to the detriment of our own physical appearance and bodily functions. Hey, on the plus, it's not all bad! Bar the dodgy continental drift that occurs on my face every summer, my acne-prone skin actually cleared up after having kids. I also used to suffer terribly from IBS – that too has gone, and for several of my friends, their endometriosis has also improved post-childbirth. Also, one of the few benefits of having twenty members of a labour ward's elbows deep in your insides is that procedures such as smear tests become a walk in the park! Zero fucks given. It's actually a nice opportunity to get out of the house and have a little lie down. Every cloud has a silver uterine lining.

There can be a lot of pressure for us womankind to 'bounce back' physically and mentally in our new postpartum lives … but as we seemingly risk weeing ourselves when we bounce, probably best we stay still, eat cake, and stick a finger up to anyone who disagrees. Right?

11

Hurty Thirty

Back in our younger days, many of us assumed that by the time we became actual grown-ups, we'd have our lives all figured out. Our careers would be high flying, romantic relationships flourishing, our Tesco Clubcard's whereabouts would be known, and there'd be no guilt associated with spending over £30 on a pair of jeans.

While you're presuming you're going to be young forever, and there's all the time in the world to achieve your dreams, life stealthily passes you by … time cruelly slipping through your fingers, as your tits slip past your belly button. So what then happens when you reach a pivotal age in adulthood and realise … you aren't where you thought you'd be? Nothing is rock and roll, everything clicks when going from seated to standing, and those milestone goals set in your teenage days have absolutely not been accomplished. Are you the only one who is now more confused than ever about the direction in which your life and décolletage are heading? Let me assure you, you most definitely are not …

Things weren't working … something was off, and it stank. Stuck in a love–hate relationship, I tried my very hardest to nurture it, but where life should have bubbled to the surface there was inactivity and an unwillingness to change. My friends were desperate for me to get online and swipe for easier options. Would I be able to throw it all away like that, though? The thought of letting the kids down was horrific … how could we tell them Mummy and Daddy failed? My husband did try, initially, but then he gave up completely. To him, it wasn't worth saving …

'Soph, I don't give a shit about the sourdough starter. Just buy a bloody Toastie Loaf!'

Welcome to 30, bitches! Artisan bread, dog walks, and garden Crocs.

I wasn't ready for it. Not at all. Fuck right off with those 'prime of your life' bullshit birthday cards. I was halfway to a free bus, and a nervous breakdown. There is a subtle mental shift as you head out of your late twenties and into your hurty thirties … creeping into that next age bracket on a local election ballot was enough to send me kicking and screaming into my next decade – downing a bottle of vodka as I went, and vomiting out of a taxi window.

Things weren't quite as expected at the point of my big milestone. The illustrious PR career that had been foretold hadn't quite materialised – mainly because it finally dawned on me that picking a profession based on your love of *Absolutely Fabulous* wasn't a sensible choice. The bosses were mean, the girls were bitchy, and I didn't even own one piece of Lacroix, sweetie! Absolutely Fuck-awful. My only career highlight was taking Andi Peters out for lunch, which was a great claim to fame but not enough to offset the lows of carting round a defrosting 'World's Biggest Fish Finger' on a press trip, brainstorming creative ideas to make tampons 'sexier', and organising events for people who liked to dress their cats up as Father Christmas. Very soon into experiencing life as a fully fledged, working grown-up, I wanted out.

Can we just take a minute, though, to appreciate how much pressure we put on kids when it comes to deciding their futures at the tender and pretty stupid age of 14? GCSE options, then A levels, followed by a rushed UCAS form filled out two hours before the submission deadline. Looking back, it was such a big decision – how was I meant to know what I wanted out of life when I couldn't even decide which outfit to wear to Yates's Wine Lodge? (It was *always* jeans and a black top ... BUT WHICH ONE? The Jane Norman halter, or the Warehouse boob tube?)

Oh, how I wish fashion decisions nowadays were this simple ... because once you arrive, on your hands and knees, at thirty's door (mostly in leopard print) you realise what a strange age bracket you now sit in for buying clothes. You're not quite young and hip, but you're also not quite old with a broken hip, and so sit in a confusing bracket that leaves you questioning whether cycling shorts will make you look cool, or like a sausage that's burst its skin. I have no idea of what is considered trendy any more – I'm highly suspicious the word 'trendy' itself is highly 'untrendy' ... Buying decisions start to hinge on practicality – items that are great for hiding various body parts, for example, rank higher than those likely to accentuate your 'fat arm' on a group photo. High heels look lovely – but how useful are they when doing the 100-metre sprint after a toddler shoplifting a Boots lipstick tester? And WHY, for the love of God, are all tops cropped? When did this creep back out of the nineties and become a thing again? T-shirts, hoodies, dressy ones for nights out – all likely to give you a chill on your kidneys. I know danger when I see it! Just a note here – mainstream online shopping past a certain age is like a toxic relationship cycle you can't quite break. It's not right for you, you think it is, but it's not – you'll spend hours of your life scrolling and crying, only to order 75 things then send 75 totally hideous and vag-skimming things back. It's time to move on.

The biggest fashion upset of them all, however, is 'mom jeans'. I want to find, and slap, the person who designed these unflattering, shapeless trousers you can tuck your tits into and then cruelly named them after child-bearing women. DO ONE! Here's the real kicker, though – as a 'mom', I look proper shit in them. THE INSULT! It only appears to be twenty-something trendsetters who can pull them off – the rest of us just look like we're applying for a motor-engineering apprenticeship three decades ago. Why do they all have large areas of material missing from the kneecap area too? Most mums will tell you that we very rarely shave above the ankle, especially when wearing jeans, so exposing three winters' worth of leg/pubic hair, and a nipple, through a seven-inch slash down the shin just isn't practical for us. I'll tell you what 'mom' jeans should actually look like … a snot-stained denim advent calendar – just endless pockets for bits of Lego, half-eaten cereal bars and wine miniatures.

Do you remember when you used to have a fairly decent social life at the weekends? One that didn't consist of jet washing a patio, cleaning cucumber jizz out of the vegetable drawer, or freezing your tits off while watching your kid's football team get spanked 26–0. Days were spent shopping with friends and having leisurely lunches while discussing outfits for that evening's drinking and debauchery. Well, hit 30 and that's just not your scene any more … Unless doing your Aldi big shop, eating ham straight out the pack while fantasising about which pyjamas you're wearing later counts? If you've got kids, clothes shopping with them should also be recategorized as a form of extreme sport. Forget skydiving and snowboarding, nothing gets the adrenaline pumping like legging it out of a changing room after a kid whose favourite game is 'run away while Mummy's half-naked'. Big shout out to the people who place little children's rides at approximately 100-metre intervals in shopping centres too, meaning you have to stop every other minute to lie out of your arse. 'Oh, Mummy doesn't have any change, sweetheart. Crying shame ...' Just a heads-up on this for anyone yet to find out for themselves, those fuckers NOW TAKE CARDS! Meaning it's going to take four hours to do a shopping trip that, if on your own, would take forty-five minutes.

Anyway, what do you need nice clothes for? Do you even go out any more? Out out, that is, and not to a friend's house at 3 p.m. for a barbecue with all your kids in tow. Doesn't really count, does it? You're always on duty, monitoring how many kids they are decking and how many Capri-Sun's they're necking. Impressive really, if they can get through one – easier to get into Fort Knox than one of those fruity bastards. *'Sip before you squeeze!'*

But while I'd love to just let loose and have a mega girls' trip to Ibiza, I'm not too sure how well this lightweight narcoleptic – who, with age, has become terrified of flying – would fare for longer than 24 hours. Also, a young person once told me the big DJs only go on to do their sets at around 4 a.m. FOUR? That can't be right ... presumably a special slot for parents whose kids get up really early? No, realistically I'm more likely to regularly visit the Isle of Wight than the White Isle ... probably in a tent ... trying not to shout at anyone who's ever come in or out of me.

Your circle of friends changes also – this is not a bad thing. Some of my absolute besties are my school mum crew, or as I like to call them 'my diamonds in the muff'. A rarity in these bitchy playground times, but my fellow forgetters of PE kits and reading books are some of the most amazing friends a girl (who has no idea when sports day is) could ever ask for. Yes, nothing beats staying in (because you're all saving for house extensions, or divorces) and chugging back gin and tonics while discussing other people's weird children, hot dads at school, and busting out some nineties and noughties tunes. As the booze and crisps flow, so do the Spice Girls and Backstreet Boys nostalgic dance routines – massively increasing the chances of injuring yourself horribly by moving too quickly in a certain direction. On a serious note, two of my friends have recently broken actual bones in their bodies from doing very little. Terrifying. One decided to do Couch To 10K and got a stress fracture that gave way when her toddler took a run up and head-butted her shins. Four months later, she's still in a leg brace and is now an unwilling participant in a challenge she did not sign up to – Couch To 10 … kg heavier. My other friend managed to snap her toe doing fuck all. FUCK ALL. Has no idea how she did it, just woke up one day with a fat foot and unable to put any weight on it. She claims it was an uncomfortable pair of shoes worn on the school run; I'm suspicious it was when she attempted to climb a lamp post after eight margaritas. My neck recently fell victim to the curse of the disintegrating ancient mummy too, after I sat up too quickly in bed turning off my alarm. Thank God Steve was home to hoist me out and tend to my needs, because I was unable to manoeuvre any of my limbs without sobbing. Him being a physio and all, I was in safe yet not overly sympathetic hands … 'I'll pull your knickers down but I'm absolutely not wiping for you!' Apparently, after I checked the small print of our wedding vows, that's not covered in the 'sickness and health' part of the contract. It took me two weeks to regain full range of movement in my neck – about the same length of time it took Steve to get over the morning after curry night.

Hypochondria is totally a thing now too! If you can break a rib sneezing or pop your hip while trying to dance along to Usher's 'Pop Ya Collar', it stands to reason that any new ailment has the potential to be fatal – causing huge panic that you, much like your invincible twenties, are history.

I found my first grey hair recently, too; it was a dark day … literally – out came the 'jet black' box dye, and I buried the fucker. Grey hair is the least of your problems, though, (unless pubic) … slower metabolism, uneven fat distribution, and skin sagginess also come knocking like the antichrist version of the Avon lady. In my twenties my figure was belting, and it really wasn't appreciated … BY ME! I ate anything (at stupid times of the night) and barely exercised, occasionally going for a run around the block and doing six sit-ups before a summer holiday. Looking back at pictures from my youth, I wish I could go back in time and slap myself. There I was looking amazing in bikinis, strappy tops and denim shorts, yet feeling horrifically self-conscious for absolutely no bloody reason. If young me could see my belly button right now, she'd be strutting about wearing bikinis daily, and rejoicing at not having to spend months of her life googling 'not too mumsy swimming costumes'. NEWSFLASH! They don't exist. They're all floral with a low-cut leg, have the structural framework of the Hoover Dam, and are thick enough to take a bullet.

A busy life, pregnancies, and a general lack of enthusiasm have resulted in the scales not quite reading how they used to fifteen years ago, either … something that occasionally cuts deep into my confidence, and love handles. Finding the motivation to exercise nowadays is just that much harder, and most nights all I actually want to do after screaming at people twelve times to use their listening ears is collapse on the sofa, eat cereal from a mug and wonder if my husband's hard of hearing. What tends to happen is that I do one brutal session (thinking it will shift 5 kg) and then wake up with the most horrific DOMS (Delayed Onset Mum Soreness) and I have to walk to school for the next four days resembling John Wayne, if he had a nasty case of thrush.

Here's a question for you. Are you even in your thirties if you haven't done any of these things: formed an emotional attachment to Joe Wicks because he's a nice man with good hair who doesn't shout at you; panic-bought ridiculous exercise equipment from a shopping channel at 3 a.m.; or signed up to a Pilates class you've only ever attended once … mainly because you farted and can't go back? Guilty of all three. Another thing about no longer being in your physical prime is that it seems to take twice the effort to burn off all those extra cupboard calories. My metabolic rate is absolutely screwed – if I eat a Twix, I gain a stone. Not fair, that, but – and it's a big but (stop it …) – I am who I am and our short lives on this planet are for living. Maybe one of the good things about getting a bit older is that you start to care a little less about your body shape. I've definitely learnt to be much kinder to myself physically and mentally. Achievable, realistic goals are the key – for example, is it possible to wear two pairs of Spanx at any one time? Probably not, so don't put yourself through it. As long I'm healthy and happy in my own skin, that's all that matters … well, that, and bread. Also, on the plus, when I'm carrying a little bit of padding it fills my wrinkles out, because that's also a thing now. Crevices so deep small woodland creatures could set up home in them. It's slow to begin with, subtle … a slight crease in your make-up that wasn't there before … then boom! Your child's sitting on your knee curiously stroking your face and asking what the lines on your forehead are. Retrospectively, a misspent youth of sun worshiping and subbing water for Apple VKs – not a great long-term beauty regime. Anyway, soaking up the rays is definitely off the agenda now because sunny days are all about washing the bedlinen on a good 60°C cycle and getting it hung on the line pronto. Weight, I'm fairly philosophical about … I feel like I get some input on that, and if I want or need to do something about it, I will. What bothers me more is Brother Nature taking my face and turning it into one of his old wrinkly, and occasionally hairy, testicles. I would honestly love to be one of these people who goes silently into the night, happy to age gracefully, but my money's on me being dragged (screaming obscenities) out of an Under 21's disco – while demanding the number of a cosmetic surgeon. I recently had a hangover pillow-line that stayed on my face for fifteen hours. FIFTEEN. It was as though my body had directed all necessary hydrating fluids away from my skin and towards my vital organs instead, leaving me looking like a Disney villain who'd just pushed my brother into a stampeding herd of buffalo. It's not just my face, though … the skin is starting to go on my décolletage (that's old-person chat for tits), and also on the back of my hands. When I was little, I used to sit for hours and pull the skin on the back of grandad's hand, then wait to see how long it would take to go back down again. MY CHILDREN NOW DO THIS TO ME. Bad times. Here's the question, though, what to do about it? Anything? Nothing? Do I really want to inject poison into myself in a bid to look constantly surprised at how shiny my forehead is? Maybe … I'm not sure. I know people my age who dabble in a bit of Botox. There are parties that spring up in the kitchens of random school mums – a friend of a friend who's offering to inject two for the price of one. It's tempting, but I'm also really scared about not being able to move my forehead because one of my biggest power moves with the kids is to raise one eyebrow and just glare. It's my only superhero skill and I'm terrified that if my face is paralysed, I'll never be able to get them to tidy their shit up off the floor.

Why do we do it to ourselves? Well, women have been trying to stave off the impending fate of ageing since the dawn of the time – it's no new phenomenon; the ancient Egyptians, however, didn't have access to Susan from school's cat's dental hygienist who has an internet qualification in aesthetics. Yep, *Death Becomes Her* just became a whole lot more accessible. Not only are cosmetic procedures more readily available nowadays, there's also no getting away from them – it seems as though our social media newsfeeds are constantly filled with the flawless faces of enhanced twenty-or thirty-somethings who have either gone to town with the fillers, or filters. None of it is real. Clever lighting, a positioning of a hip, or an arch of a spine, and a hundred discarded snaps later the perfect picture is finally ready to be uploaded and adored by the masses. The dick-pic takers really need to take note. I personally have nothing against the Kardashian contingency; in some ways, I feel their dominance over the media for years has actually helped to transform a beauty industry that at one point thought the only body type commercially acceptable was an emaciated one. The problem, however, with us mere mortals attempting to 'Keep up with the Klones' is that they are predominately smoke and mirrors. Beautiful women made even more beautiful by an army of make-up artists, hairdressers and stylists. It's a dangerous and unachievable ideology that many of us fall into the trap of believing, and so let feelings of inadequacy and insecurity creep into our heads. Without a doubt, I'm so guilty of not appreciating that ageing is actually a privilege not all of us can bank on. Our faces have tales to tell – about the places we've been, the people we've met, our love, laughter, and pain ... Maybe one day we'll all feel comfortable enough in our skin to liberate those lines and let them proudly share their stories with the world ... and maybe, just maybe, I'll let my face speak a thousand words ... Heads-up, it will probably just shout, 'I SUNBATHED TOO MUCH AND MY KIDS NEVER FUCKING SLEPT!'

With the arrival of my mid-thirties came a fairly large milestone in Steve's and my relationship – our ten-year wedding anniversary. Nowadays, 20-year-olds aren't thinking about signing up to a life of commitment, they're thinking about signing up to *Love Island*. It's all about the blue tick, huns. I'm actually very proud of us getting to a decade of marriage, and that's not because I didn't ever think, pre-vows, we wouldn't make it ... when I said 'until death us do part' I meant it. There's no getting away from me, even from six feet under – I'm still going to hang around and make sure he's not remarrying anyone hotter. No, I'm proud of us because the past ten years haven't all been plain sailing, jam-packed full of romance, and rampant bonking. Married life is tough; it takes hard work, compromise, and a sense of realism. Being 25 when we got hitched, our first few years of marriage coincided with some pretty amazing life experiences – endless nights out, travelling the world, being able to leave the house with just my phone and a lipstick. Then our thirties crashed down upon us … we took on a big mortgage, fired out a couple of kids, and were fully submerged into the grind of 9–5. We realised we were stuck in a rut of routine, responsibilities, and regurgitation – mainly mine; my drinking ability was shot to shit after pregnancy. I'm not going to sugar-coat it – there are a lot of changes that occur within a relationship after being with someone for that length of time. Losing the thrill of the chase is a big one … those once ever-present phero'moans and animalistic urges to rip each other's clothes off the minute you get home from work dissipate slightly over time, replaced by a need to know what's for dinner instead. You go from horny hyenas to hungry hippos. Throw kids into that mix and sometimes it's just not practical to have a shag on the kitchen worktop when there's a two-year-old smearing Weetabix all over it. It's not that you don't fancy your partner any more, it's just that the stresses and strains of everyday life can take over … and when you've been pawed all day by a little person, sometimes the last thing you want is to be pawed by a big one. 'No offence, babe, but don't lay one finger on me – especially if it's sticky.'

Interesting fact of the day, and something I discovered in the baby-making process, is that a woman's libido heavily depends on where she's at in her menstrual cycle, which makes total sense. When you're ovulating, you're on heat; when you're not, you'd rather watch Netflix and chill ... on your own ... in a different room ... in flannel pyjamas. Brother Nature didn't think that one through, did he? Too late now, fucker. It does make me feel slightly guilty, though, that I don't always have the same sex drive as my husband ... but not guilty enough to stop lying about the actual length of my period. 'Still on the dregs, babe, sorry!'

Another change in the relationship centres around the level of importance you put on significant dates. Take Valentine's Day and anniversaries. Remember the early throes of a coupling when love and lust are still at full pelt? Roses are red, violets are blue and they at least remembered a bastard card for you. For our first Christmas, Steve bought me a diamond bracelet. Diamonds! Cut to ten years down the line and for our wedding anniversary, he suggested we didn't 'do' presents and instead finally pursue our ultimate mid-thirties fetish fantasy ... getting the extension done. Little did I know, we were actually entering into an awkward eighteen-month, incredibly dirty three-way with a builder who had horrific dietary fibre intake issues. So, there was a verbal agreement to not exchange gifts for our tenth wedding anniversary but, like most of womankind, despite saying I didn't *want* a present, I still expected to *get* one. Men, just a heads-up here – when a woman says she doesn't want a present, it just might be a lie. What we're actually saying when our lips appear to be mouthing 'OK, that's fine' is 'I want an eternity ring the size of my head'. It's all just one big mind-bending test. You should also know that even though you've specifically requested for us not to get you anything, we will still buy you a present ... mainly to lord it over you in all future arguments until the end of time.

Do you know what the official gift for ten years of lights-off, socks-on loving is? Bearing in mind a lot of us get a diamond just for agreeing to marriage in the first place? Tin. That's right, your long-service award is canned goods that'll outlive an apocalypse. Despite the advance warning, I was still dreaming of some platinum-set bling and was of course more than happy to get him something he really wanted too … but as you can't get blow jobs in a tin (sadly just hand jobs), I settled on some lovely artisan beers. The big day arrived, as did the exchange of presents … he opened his beers, and I opened … SWEET FA! The rest of the day was then spent thinking of different ways to do him in with pale ales (nearly all resulted in death by severely itchy yeast infection). I did get one present, though: the ability to win every argument for the next fifty years – some may agree that, really, it was actually the best gift of all.

Sometimes we squabble, have totally unrealistic expectations, and annoy the hell out of each other; sometimes, possibly, we may independently pine for a bit of our younger and more exciting lives back – but isn't that just marriage? You are two individual people who sign up for a lifetime of love and living together, and over that course, things won't always run smoothly – how can they? In fact, I'm always heavily suspicious of people who say they never fight with their partner – it's healthy to be able to tell your ride or die that they're being a colossal dickhead. Steve and I definitely are not the same people we were in our carefree twenties. Fragments of our former selves remain, but we've grown, adapted, and become stronger. We're a unit, a force to be reckoned with, and the biggest champions for each other's causes. Annoyingly, he's ageing better – like a fine wine. He's a total fox. I'm ageing like a half-drunk bottle of Prosecco – a bit dry, leaves a funny taste in your mouth, and rapidly losing fizz. Not in his eyes, though; as long as I've still got a pulse, I'm all good. I'll know our love is dead the minute I bend over to put something in a cupboard and he doesn't hip thrust me from behind. He might not be 'The Rock' but I'll tell you what, he's my rock – an unflappable, level-headed yin to my yang and I wouldn't swap him for the world. But maybe for a shirtless, dripping wet Channing Tatum holding a big fuck-off diamond eternity ring ... Joke! Take out Channing and add in Chris Hemsworth. On a serious note, in our ten years of marriage, I've taken the bin out all of twice. He's not going anywhere.

So yes, things are not *quite* what I thought they'd be, but in a way ... that's good! I've actually achieved different goals to the ones I set out in my younger days, and arguably I've actually done more with my life than 18-year-old me predicted – I bloody created it, TWICE! Also, I think we can all agree, anyone who thinks it's RAD to use black kohl liner on their lips should not be put in charge of determining the success of anyone's future. So yes, finding a perfectly ripe avocado is one of the greatest highlights of my week, my Pinterest search history is full of wooden flooring options, I'm concerned about the black spots on my pear tree, and I have *MasterChef* on series link. This is life now, and I'm semi-accepting of my fate. Also, it's not until you're approaching 40 that you realise what a monumental twat you were for worrying about turning 30. I might not understand fashion, be able to stand in heels for longer than twelve minutes, or get up from a chair without making a strange wheezing noise, but I am in the prime of my life – Amazon prime ... they've got some cracking deals on non-stick pans.

Growing up isn't all bad, and on the plus, at least your drinking ability increases with age, and your hangovers decrease ...

PSYCHE!

PTO ...

12

From Cradle to Rave

There comes an age when things start to become less regular, dry up, and eventually ... stop all together. It's a difficult time in life, and one that takes a huge amount of adjustment. The good news, however, is you're not going through it on your own – friends of a similar age are also feeling the unwanted side effects of 'the change' ... to your social life.

Past 30 and with kids constantly consuming all aspects of your existence, frequent nights out, sadly, become a thing of the past – unless bombing it out to a twenty-four-hour supermarket at 1 a.m. for Calpol, or fondant icing, counts? No? That's cool, I was asking for a friend anyway. There's a part of you that mourns the person you once were ... a crop-top wearing, glitter in hair, dancing until dawn tequila downer – but there's also a slightly bigger part that enjoys elasticated loungewear, living vicariously through 20-year-old reality stars, and doing shots ... of Pringles straight from the tub.

Opportunities to see friends and reclaim that shred of your former self are, more often than not, few and far between – especially when surgically attached to vulnerable humans who without you wouldn't be able source food, find a single thing, or wipe their own arses. In these instances, get a divorce and move on. The closest you've been to a good dance was at the kids' football club's Christmas party, where there may, or may not, have been a round of 4 p.m. shots and an unfortunate twerking incident between yourself and one of the coaches. So when the opportunity for a PROPER girls' night arises, and all the stars align, resulting in fifteen women managing to coordinate a date in their diaries for a Saturday two years in the future, it absolutely has to be seized. Or does it? Despite looking forward to a mammoth mum piss-up for months, and it being the highlight of your WhatsApp group chats, when the actual date looms, so do those second thoughts … It's Saturday night and you feel bad about abandoning your favourite small people … Ant and Dec. More importantly, what the bloody hell are you going to wear? As lovely as it is to leave the house in clothing not contaminated with snot, beans, or the bodily fluids of others, you're not left with many options that aren't maternity leggings, despite not having been pregnant in the past three years. As previously mentioned, the world of online shopping, especially after a certain age, can be a shambolic experience that may leave you questioning whether Boohoo was named after the emotional response evoked in customers over the age of 30. And don't forget Forever 21, a shop created to constantly remind you of being closer to Fucking 41

Settling on 'jeans and a nice top', and with Spanx kicking off your IBS (Itchy Bits Syndrome), it's time to tipsily apply winged eyeliner that after several attempts is alarmingly close to your hairline, before escaping from the arse-wiping hellmouth (mini bottle of Prosecco in hand) into the waiting taxi outside. That said, you do still have your phone on, though, just in case ... you want to Instagram the shit out of your pretty, double-washed-hair and unfamiliar with flattering angles double-chinned self. #FeltCuteMightVomLater. Already in the cab, and halfway to being totally leathered, are three of your mates who have demanded the poor driver uses his DAB radio as a low-budget karaoke machine. 'Dave, Dave, Dave, Dave, Dave ... you got anything by Olly Murs?' Dave does not. He hates his life, us, and blokes who wear loafers without socks. He also does not take kindly to you playing with his knob. 'Love, I've already told you – stop messing with the stations!' Dumped kerbside, and resembling a bunch of day-release prisoners who are about to ruin their chances of parole, you've forgotten all about those pre-outing jitters because an 'out of sight, out of mind' mentality has kicked in and you're officially that mum who's binned off the kids and wants to get fucked up.

It's a tricky one, though, because you're also that mum who drinks two gin and tonics, has a fight with her stairs, and then vomits on her shoes. Here's the thing about mums on a night out – we do have a *slight* tendency to go a *little* bit WILD. Potentially it's the giddiness of leaving the house without taking rice cakes, or maybe it's the Spanx cutting off the blood supply to our heads ... either way, David Attenborough needs to get himself set up behind the wheely bins of a chicken shop.

'Here we see the commonly spotted 'shit-faced' mum. Seldom separated from her young, tonight she can be seen necking twelve bottles of Prosecco, fishing control pants out of her arse crack, and pole dancing ... against a policeman.'

We all have that one friend, don't we, who can't quite take the bubbles, has seen *Showgirls* too many times, and thinks she's the dog's bollocks gyrating to Justin Timberlake. 'I'm bringing sexy back!' No, you're not Carol, OK? You're 42, you work in accounts. All you're bringing back is your stress incontinence ... calm yourself! But Carol will not be calmed because she is a zebra, recently released from captivity, and she, along with her vajazzle dazzle, is NEVER going back!

'Feet bloodied from high-hooves, and limping like their postpartum days ... it has been a treacherous migration from child-infested habitats to the plain's most exotic of watering holes ... Slug and Lettuce. Bitterly disappointed at not being asked for identification by the bearded bison protecting the entrance, they locate additional members of the herd using a call sign unique only to the female species – a series of high-pitched screams and shrieks, followed by limb flapping. The oldest mummals in the vicinity by a clear ten years, it's time to drown their sorrows with a few more bottles of the establishment's finest Prosecco, or as they'll be calling it in the morning ... prosicco.'

With the drinks and laughter flowing, glimmers of the woman you once were begin to shine through and it feels glorious. This is amazing, and liberating! Why don't you do this more often?! Then your phone rings ...

'For the hundredth time, babe, if you need to put the grill on, turn the dial to G. Is that the kids crying in the background? Have you not fed them yet? It's 8.30!'

Blocking images of cremated chicken nuggets from your mind, it's time to hit the dance floor with the girls and bring the joint down with your sexy moves ... your hip joint, that is. Slut-dropping after you've had kids – NOT advisable, you do not have the necessary core or pelvic strength for it. In your head, you're Nicole Sherzinger, but in reality, much less Pussycat Doll, much more pissy-cat doll. In the process, you will have also ruptured a hamstring and won't be able to walk without a limp for two months. After several ill-advised rounds of sambuca, sixty deleted 'fat arm' photos, and being told to get off the tables by the management, it's time to call it a night … it's 9.05 p.m.

The biggest night out in a mum's social calendar, however, has to be … a hen party! Like a normal night but ten times the debauchery, and double the amount of thonged men flapping their giant floppy appendages in your face while you're trying to have an in-depth conversation with your bestie about organic washing powder. Female strippers, I get … absolutely. Us gals tend to look a teeny bit more appealing in a sequinned thong. But a guy called Greg, with dodgy tats, and an eyebrow piercing, descending from the ceiling like a scantily clad disco Spider-Man and then offering to shoot his special web all over your face … is that sexy? I'm not so sure … the jury, much like his cock, is out. Thank goodness that on my own bachelorette friends knew how particular I am when it comes to the penises I let near my face – no stranger's knob goblin shall pass until it's had a thorough DBS check – that's Dick Balls Scrotum. You know when a daddy-long-legs flies at you unexpectedly and you panic bitch-slap it away while standing on a chair screaming for help? My exact reaction to a male lap dance. I'd be more turned on if the dude arrived with a pack of root vegetable crisps and some guacamole. It's the only way a parsnip's getting dipped in anything.

It used to really annoy me that men went on 'stag' parties like a bunch of proud, horned, majestic beasts, while us women got labelled as a bunch of scatty, flapping chickens. That was until I tried to cross a road with twenty other drunk females dripping in penis paraphernalia and immediately I understood the characterisation. 'Girls! Everyone look left, look right, look left again … wait for that bus and twelve other vehicles to start heading directly at us … and cross!' Why did the hen party cross the road? To get flattened by a double-decker bus while dressed as a bunch of slutty nuns.

That said, one of my favourite parts of a hen party is the obligatory and morally demeaning fancy dress. No matter the theme, we always find a way to sex it up, don't we? Apart from that one hen who doesn't get the memo and arrives in full habit and nana shoes while everyone else looks like Madonna circa 'Like a Prayer'. On my friend Helen's hen party, the theme was 'characters from your childhood'. There we all were, dressed as sex-pot Little Red Riding Hoods, or Bo Beep in a suspender belt and fuck-me boots looking for her blow-up sheep, and then there was my friend Amy, who turned up as the Wicked Witch of the West, head to toe in green paint and leaving little trails of green behind her as though she had gonorrhoea.

There really is something about a hen party that sends normally very rational and sensible women absolutely delirious with excitement. The bad behaviour I've seen on these ritualistic celebrations would make grown men cry, and normally some of the worst offenders are the mums. We just don't get out all that often, do we? When you don't know when it might happen again, it's always best to err on the side of caution and make the most of the opportunity while you can – and if that means spending a night in the cells because you stole the helmet of the policeman you were pole dancing against and then dry-humped his leg as he was attempting to retrieve it, so be it. Hen parties generally make for the more interesting nights because you won't always necessarily know all of the ladies in attendance. Outside of your own friendship-circle breakaway group, there'll be the bride's relatives, potentially her in-laws, oddball work colleagues who've been invited out of politeness, and of course the worst group of all … the non-bill-splitters. Eugh. Thanks to them, a task that should be a simple two-minute calculation turns into something more reminiscent of a *University Challenge* tiebreaker. 'I only had a starter for ten … quid!' If ever you've felt a bit miffed at not being asked to be a bridesmaid, take a lot of solace in knowing it's officially the worst job in the world – effectively a debt collector in a beauty queen sash who's responsible for the lives of twenty inebriated souls, all while being £100 down because it was easier than trying to work out who'd shortchanged the group. The last hen party I went on perfectly sums up the majority of these occasions … classy to begin with, but come 9.30 p.m., after aimlessly wandering the streets for an hour, everyone's standing in a very questionable nightspot called Shades (CHAR-DAZE, though, innit?) wondering what the funny smell is. By 10 p.m. you'll be life coaching other drunk women in the toilets, while keeping a breastfeeding friend company as she hand-milks herself. Returning from the loos, several members of the group will have lost the ability to speak in coherent sentences, yet are still capable of a word-perfect rendition of S Club 7's 'Reach'. You also seem to have acquired a crying girl called Donna, who keeps asking to borrow your brush, and can't find any of her mates. It's very loud too, so loud you can't hear each other speak – you'll have a twenty-minute shouty conversation with your bestie discussing that very matter, while also pondering why it's so very dark? Now, dodgy nightclubs are generally dark for two reasons – the first of which is so that you don't see whatever the heck is responsible for the vommy smell. The second, so you don't notice the pack of sweaty middle-aged hyenas lurking in the 'VIP' roped-off corner, who are already drawing up their tactical advance strategy. Unfortunately, hens have the ability to attract every knobhead within a twelve-mile radius. There you all are, dancing in your satanic-cult circle, worshiping the pagan goddess of handbags, and being led in a chorus of 'Single Ladies' by your penis-head-band-wearing high priestess, when from out of nowhere, bam! You're surrounded …

'Unsure of the hens' defensive capabilities, the cackling male hyenas opt to send the weakest member of the pack forward first, to test the waters and their receptiveness at being joined by six greasy males – all of which work in IT. With sixteen pints of Stella Artois under his belt, Phill makes his move … Perspiring heavily from his face, armpits and groin area, he has opted to salsa-dance his way into the middle of the flock, in an attempt to wear them down with his snake hips and matted chest fur. It is a mistake. Immediately detecting the threat of a drunken dickhead, the brood instinctively changes formation, blocking his advances with a series of wing-jabbing motions and disgruntled clucks. With the rest of the attention-starved hyenas separating in order to cover more ground, it's time for the alpha, Mike, to show his scavenging clan how it's done. Resembling a sweatier version of Mr Tumble, he hip-thrusts his way towards the pissed-off poultry, unaware that danger is afoot for this brazen and arrogant predator. With absolutely none of the hens wanting to see what's inside his spotty ball bag, they are prepared for his gyrating advances, sending Donna, now bleeding heavily from her foot, towards him at full speed brandishing a Smirnoff Ice and menacingly squawking at him to 'CLUCK OFF!'. Their pride dented, literally – Donna lobbed the bottle – they retreat … home to their wives, and four young offspring. They may be carnivores, but they're definitely closer to a bunch of cocks.'

Of course, the holy grail of all hen parties, to a lot of mums, is the foreign one. The possibility of hopping on a plane and experiencing a weekend of boozy hedonism in the sun WITHOUT CHILDREN is just too much for our CBeebies-addled minds to take. No inflatable unicorns, no 20 kg luggage allowance of snacks, and no responsibility?! YES PLEASE! My problem is that I'm at an age where a lot of my friends are either married, or they don't want to be, which is fine, I totally respect their selfish decisions – but it does mean opportunities for these highly joyful rarities are becoming less and less. I'm starting to look at people I know and their relationships very questioningly … are they really that happy? Will they make it? Am I a bad person for casually suggesting re-marrying when husband-bitching is happening, and uploading dating apps onto their phone while sliding a holiday brochure into their tissue-clenching hands? Granted, it might be a tad extreme but those who don't have children will never understand the excitement of the free pass that is *needing* to go abroad for a weekend. They can just leave the country whenever they please. 'Might pop off to an adults-only hotel in Mykonos this Friday!' Good for you – the only time my kids will be letting me visit an adults-only residence will be when I'm 70 and they're putting me in a home.

A hen party 1300 miles away is the only justifiable way I can push my mum guilt to one side for two days, let my newly combed-for-nits hair down, and leave my husband to microwave fish fingers. So when the 'high school crew' WhatsApp group goes off and it's a picture of an engagement ring … well, the excitement is insurmountable! You don't even offer a congratulatory response, just a straight to the point 'WHERE ARE WE GOING ON THE HEN PARTY?!' Expedia's already loading, you're googling 'where's hot in March', and then comes the bride-to-be's response … 'I was thinking of a nice country house in The Cotswolds …' WHAT?! It takes all the restraint in the world to stop yourself from leaving the group, defriending her on Facebook and smashing some shit up. 'HOW COULD SHE DO THIS TO ME?!' The situation is made worse by the fact your other half is off on the stag do, and they're going to fucking Vegas. So while you're doing a flower-arranging class with a woman named Xanthe, and sitting through a game of Mr & Mrs where the mother of the bride has to listen to her daughter's favourite sexual position, he's off watching Calvin Harris live, tanning to the max, and spunking all the joint account money in strip clubs. The outrage.

One thing is for certain, no matter where you spend your mums' night out, the end result is pretty much always the same – a dodgy chicken shop, a friend in A&E, and deep child-birth-style breathing in the back of a taxi so as not to let your knock-off KFC fly straight back out of your mouth.

Personally, I have a massive issue when it comes to judging my own li*mum*tations. When surrounded by fellow overexcited females I become far too giddy and get caught up in the moment, forgetting a) Sambuca may taste like Gaviscon, but it is not, b) my stomach's constitution is as weak as my pelvic floor, and c) I HAVE CHILDREN. Crawling out of the cab, one stiletto in hand and spilling my chips all up the driveway, it truly is a sight to behold. Sir David would have a field day …

'Having spent twenty minutes trying to open her front door with a car key fob, and shouting obscenities at a neighbour's judgemental cat, she is eventually let in by her eye-rolling mate. On the hunt for sustenance, she mauls six packs of Pom-Bears, sliced ham straight from the pack, and two crumpets she mistakenly thinks are covered in Nutella, but is actually Marmite. She is, however, yet to face her biggest nemesis … the stairs. There's Everest, K2, Kilimanjaro, and then there's the flight of steps connecting the downstairs of her

house to the upstairs. An underdog with the eye of a tiger, who must first find a way out from underneath her own dog, she rises up to the challenge of her rival and eventually makes it to the summit. Collapsing into bed fully dressed, but minus a shoe, only one final task remains – pinning a less than impressed mate to the edge of the bed using only the power of stagnant alcohol and yeast-extract breath. At 3 a.m. comes the unmistakable churning sensation of bad life choices. She hugs the toilet bowl as litres of regurgitated crump-bears and prosicco explode from within. Denial of her lack of ability to know one's own limits has absolutely convinced her the torrents of bodily fluid escaping via her nasal passage is due to food poisoning, not mixing the grape with the grain followed by a porn star martini, and several shots. Despite wailing loudly and expressing a fear of being close to death, her sleeping mate does not wake, leaving this highly regretful female to suffer alone … until 6 a.m., that is, when two small people burst into the room like someone's fired them out of a very fucking loud and cheery canon.'

You cannot convince me otherwise of this – parenting with a hangover is punishment for sins committed in a previous life. Even if Steve is home, and is perfectly capable of sorting out the kids' million and one requests, they will still, purposefully, go out of their way to come and find me with my head down a toilet and ask me to wipe their arses. The morning after the night before is felt heavily among your fellow co-conspirators too. The once exuberant, giddy, 'Larry Largepants' group chat is filled with regret, shame and upwards of forty-seven vomiting emojis. What was everyone thinking? A vegetarian mum is beside herself because she woke up to find the remains of a partially mauled doner kebab in her bra, another has three broken ribs and a traffic cone in her front garden, and one thought she was sexting her husband in the cab on the way home but accidentally sent a picture of her left nipple to her in-laws via the 'family' WhatsApp group.

After chewing on a piece of dry toast for half an hour, and cradling a full-fat Coke with the love and affection of a mother holding a newborn baby, it's time to steel yourself for the worst fate that could be bestowed upon the hungover species … fucking swimming lessons. Hot, sweaty, wet, humid, verucca hell – it's your turn and not even the completely empty promise of a sexual favour can convince your partner to swap with you. Torn between not wanting your children to drown at sea, and not wanting to die in a sea of your own vomit, it's a tough hour out of the house that impacts everyone's emotional and physical well-being. With sambuca-laced sweat dripping out of every pore on your shaking body, trying to wrestle a resisting and clammy child into a pair of jeans is not going well. DENIM? Pure madness, woman!

On leaving the pool, a message pings on your phone from a fellow hanging mum asking what time you'll be arriving at the party later. WHAT PARTY? Fuck. The day is a gift that keeps on giving. Speaking of gifts, you have nothing to offer a six-year-old girl apart from a cautionary tale about responsible drinking and knowing your own limits. Two hours later, in a church hall, ears bleeding from the screams of crying children who haven't won a plastic medal from creepy Disco Dan, the situation has gone from bad to worse. Having to rein in kids completely smacked off their tits on sugar, and as a result are stabbing their friends with shivs they've crafted out of party hats, all you can think about is your next fix of beige salty carbs and what you're going to have to offer your other half in order to get them to do a McDonald's run …

Once the kids are in bed, an hour earlier than planned thanks to their inability to tell the time, I always collapse on the sofa and evaluate where it all went so horribly wrong. After much contemplating, the conclusion is that I'm too old for this shit, and I'm NEVER drinking EVER again. Well, until next time … but definitely no prosicco … well maybe only one glass … or two … but definitely not a whole bottle … or bottles … Probably.

13

The Fun Mum

Do you remember when you were a kid, and your evenings/weekends/school holidays consisted of maybe going to your mate's house, youth club, or getting dragged round the supermarket with your parents to do a big shop? That was it, our childhood entertainment. Man, our folks had it easy. Nowadays, a new parenting species has evolved … born from a combination of personal aspirations, maternal guilt, an inability to say no, and a social media inferiority complex – she is 'The Fun Mum'. An all-singing (lessons), all-dancing (classes), money-haemorrhaging powerhouse who spends what little spare time she has trying to prove to her kids (and self) that Mummy is actually an absolute riot. From giving up Saturday mornings to stand, hungover, on a muddy football pitch, to making sure in the holidays her SHIT is well and truly together (that's School Holiday Itinerary Timetable), her work of keeping her children occupied 24/7 is never done … The 'Fun Mum' can be easily identified by the following personality traits/flaws …

Idealism

What could be more fun than a good old-fashioned walk in the great outdoors? An easy and cost-effective way of getting kids out of the house to do some exercise, all while enjoying some quality time together as a family. HA! Firstly, it can take upwards of an hour from deciding you're going on a walk to actually leaving the house. In that time, a whole host of tomfoolery and dicking about will have taken place, because with my children especially, it's a fate worse than going to the supermarket.

'Eugh! A walk? Why do we have to do that?'

'Because it's healthy, sweetheart, and it's what I see all the other families who live on our road doing – with smiles on their faces, a football in their hands, and a sense of smugness that cripples my parenting inferiority complex.'

'Can I play Pokémon GO on your phone?'

Once you've located shoes, coats, a doll's pram to push, a very specific piece of Lego, and emptied bladders and bowels, along with your silent screams into a cushion, you open the door and … it's raining. Of course it is. If you are actually lucky enough to make it out, several things are bound to happen:

1. Five minutes into the excursion, the scooters they insisted on bringing will no longer be required, leaving you to carry them (spinning around and smashing into your ankles), along with a child on your hip, for the remainder of the outing.
2. The pace at which you are moving is so incredibly slow your sports watch no longer detects a pulse. Are you dead? Not physically, but your soul has moved on to a better place.

3. There'll be a fight over the bringing home of a stick. It's absolutely not coming back with you.*
4. Someone will step in dog shit.
5. Spurred on by the smell, a child will then also need a shit. The only option is a 'nature poo' which doesn't seem quite as charming as its more socially acceptable cousin, the 'nature wee', especially on the driveway of an elderly couple who are looking out of the window to see what the commotion is. You're forced to pick it up with a wet-wipe and a leaf – there is not one single bin in sight for the remainder of your outing.
6. It will take three hours to walk around your block. You feel like JLo – you always know where you came from … 0.4 miles from your front door.

Heroism

Soft. Play. Two small words that strike fear into the heart of any veteran parent. Trips to these establishments are much like paying your taxes – painful, and unavoidable. I'm always torn between wanting to wear my kids out, and not wanting to spend three hours in a louder and smellier version of Hades. Generally speaking, it's a rainy-day, last-resort move. The playground is awash with water, and menacing teenagers on bikes, so you're left with little option other than to say those fateful yet magical words out loud. 'Who wants to go to soft play?' In that moment, though, you're a hero! Fun Mum for the win! Even though they want to go, getting them out of the house and into the car is akin

* It will live outside your front door for the next six months.

to herding piss-taking sheep. By the time you've arrived, the sun is out and cracking the flags, but it's too late – you've promised and there's no backsies.

After trying to blag the smallest of the kids as being a year younger than they actually are, in order to save a quid, it's time to run through the very first rule of Soft Play Club – NEVER eat anything you find on the floor. Next up – don't climb up the slide, unless you want to be taken out by a shrieking and statically charged mum in go-faster leggings. And no more than one person on the trampoline at any time otherwise the hard-as-nails woman behind the counter will implode. That's it! Fly free, my pretties, and try to avoid dubious puddles and squished baked beans in *The Crystal Maze*'s most notorious and dangerous sector … the 'Bacteria Zone'. If you've managed to hoodwink a friend into coming with you, it's a nice opportunity to grab a coffee and not be able to hear a word they're saying – there's something about the acoustics of all soft-play centres that guarantees you leaving with scream-induced tinnitus. While you're chinwagging and sporadically flinching, the kids will have given you the slip – prompting your heart to drop through your stomach because … you'll have to fucking go in after them! WHY, GOD? WHY? To make the situation better, of course, you're not wearing socks. Praying the brown sticky thing attached to a heel is in fact a raisin, you find them … in the bastard ball pit, being assaulted by a 12-year-old with a mullet and an overarm bowl that would put Freddie Flintoff to shame. It's the ultimate test of how much you love your child – leave them to lose an eye, or get on in there and risk tetanus? Diving in like David Hasselhoff, it's the proudest moment of your parenting career until … you start to slowly drown … sinking down towards the faeces, crumbs and discarded plasters. This is the end. You don't have the core strength to get yourself out of it. What a bloody way to go. Then all of a sudden, a hand has fished you out and you're alive!

Thanking 1980s Freddie for his gallantry, it's time to exit via the highly dignified elbow-smashing, friction-burning curly slide.

One of the worst things to have ever happened to me on a soft-play outing involved one of my children overindulging in Fruit Shoots before climbing to the third 'gluttony punishing' circle of Dante's hell. It was here, on the rope bridge, that said child unfortunately lost control of their bladder, sending a waterfall of wee cascading like Niagara Falls down through not one, not two, but three layers of play equipment and drenching all children in its path. I'm not sure whether it makes the story better, or worse, to say we'd actually hired the place out for a birthday party so knew all of the children affected by this terrible tragedy. Needless to say, on all the photos, there were some very PISSed-off looking children.

After they've wolfed down some fish fingers, added a few more beans to the carpet, and had a shit-fit because having paid a tenner for them to get in you refuse to shell out any more money on an electric ride that'll last thirty seconds, it's time to extract them from the premises. It's like trying to convince a drunk person to leave a nightclub at kicking out time – there's windmilling, shoes being tossed in the air, and a last-ditch run back inside before security catches up with them. They eventually leave, sobbing, shoeless, under an arm, and with a whole pack of Cadbury's buttons shoved in their gob. Once home, there's just the small matter of disinfecting them at a distance and waiting up to seventy-two hours to see what bug they're going to come down with.

Ambition

Ahhh, the road trip … AKA 'the highway to yell...ing.' A lot. What could possibly be more fun than spending upwards of two hours in a hot and airless car with children who have no concept of time, and the patience of a teenage boy during his first sexual encounter? 'NO, WE ARE NOT NEARLY THERE YET!' And once you have kids, it becomes very apparent how hugely flawed the driving test process is. You might be able to reverse around a corner, but can you do it while offspring are clawing each other's eyes out in the back seat, asking you to look at a scab on their toe, and twatting you round the head with a balloon? If you haven't yelled 'DO YOU WANT MUMMY TO CRASH THE CAR AND KILL US ALL?!' are you even really a parent? It's pretty much a given that every car journey, accompanied by children, will go down like this …

1. *Boredom.* This will kick in within six feet of your house. You can still see your front door and they'll be whingeing about wanting to get out and go for a walk.
2. *Hunger.* They've eaten their body weight in Cheerios before they left and have consumed enough car snacks to feed a family of six for a week, yet they're still peckish. You've been on the road for ten minutes.
3. *Games.* I-spy in a car moving at 70 mph, with a child who only operates in colours, leaves you desperately attempting to guess something brown they saw potentially over an hour ago. 'Is it a tree? Mummy's hair? A field? Your teddy bear?' Of course it's not, it's the previous day's 'nature poo.'

4. *Questions.* Driving in sheets of rain past speeding lorries in tiny, narrow lanes seems to be a great time to answer very specific questions about life and death that you just don't have the answers for.
5. *Singalongs.* Having been through all the classics on repeat, for HOURS, you're forced to get creative by verse 309 of 'Old MacDonald'. 'The Indominus Rex goes rah, rah, rah …'
6. *Devices.* Hoarse from singing about the weirdest farm in all the land, you foolishly hand over an iPad, tablet, or similar – just for ten minutes of peace. What harm could it do?
7. *Vomit.* It's everywhere, and everyone is screaming. Breakfast milk has curdled into cottage cheese, the child who hasn't been sick has partially digested and incredibly 'non-cheery' cereal in their hair, and you're stuck in a traffic jam – at least thirty miles from the nearest services. Nothing says you've been on a road trip like using a toothbrush to scrub chunks out of a seat-belt buckle.
8. *Incontinence.* It takes a BRAVE parent to call the bluff of someone with a bladder the size of a walnut, and who has previous for defecating on pensioners' doorsteps. Having got them to the service station in the nick of time, you hear 'I don't need to go any more, Mummy!' Furious, you take the opportunity to spend a penny – only for them to announce, in their loudest voice possible, 'Mummy, your front bottom looks like a hamster!' Back on the road, ten minutes later … 'MUMMY! I need a wee!'
9. *Violence.* Everyone's had enough but for the siblings in the back – one's had the audacity to look at the other one 'in a funny way' and it has caused a

gladiator fight to the death. While it's going down, all you can silently and wistfully scream in your head is 'ARE WE NEARLY THERE YET?'

Open-mindedness

Family festivals – something I entirely blame Instagram for. Trendy-looking families, in their Hunter wellies, faces adorned with dolphin-killing glitter, all living their best lives dancing around to hedonistic music in sun-drenched wheat fields. It all looks so idyllic, so inspirational, so … staged. This I learned the hard way. About two years ago I got a real bee in my bonnet about not being a 'fun mum'. My worry was that in years to come the kids would all be standing round my grave, colour coordinated and in height order, potentially wishing I'd been more of a hoot while in the land of the living – the kind of mum, perhaps, you'd see on social media taking their children to fashionable and tick-filled fields. Still feeling a bit bad from over-egging our most recent fun day out to 'Food World' (Asda), I decided to bite the bullet, dig out some clothing with fringing and face my biggest challenge yet as a mum … not Lyme disease… Portaloos. Prior to kids, I most definitely wasn't a festival kind of person, but, guilted into it by the #MakingMemories crowd, I thought it was time to pop my cherry and roll around in the highly Instagrammable hay. What a legend.

Festivals can be made or broken by the weather; so it's incredibly fortunate here in England we're renowned for our predictable and blistering summers. We'd literally just stepped out of the car when the heavens opened. Entering the turnstiles, piss-wet through, we were immediately set upon by someone in a high-vis. 'Would you like to buy a £3 programme to see what's happening today?' Sorry, what now? The tickets cost £70 and we have to pay *extra* for a programme? I already knew what was happening – a big fat rip-off. Then, the children clapped eyes on the inflatable version of Disneyland, with less public liability insurance and more verrucas. 'Can we go on Mummy?'

'Of course, sweetheart! Wait … A tenner per child, for thirty minutes?!' At that point, the penny dropped that we'd spent the best part of a hundred quid to stand in a field, overseeing *Total Wipeout* in the rain, and welcoming the onset of hypothermia with open arms. Tell you what you don't see on Instagram – shit fairground rides, a decrepit donkey, a box of ten greasy donuts, and a child throwing up all over themselves on the way home. LIES. ALL LIES!

Fearlessness

Theme parks always seem like a great idea, in theory, until you get there and you realise the theme of the park is … queuing. Eardrums already bleeding from the journey's constant backseat whinge, it's comforting to know you have another six hours of 'are we nearly there yet' ahead of you … before every ride. For small children, the concept of waiting a long time for something that'll last less than a minute is not easy to get their heads around, and is a nice lesson for some adults too. Every ride you queue up for, without exception, by the time you get to the front, the kids need a wee. When you actually manage to get them on the thing, they scream the whole way round – not from enjoyment but because they didn't like it/it was too fast/not fast enough/they couldn't sit at the front/the wind changed. One of my biggest parenting failures to date involved my then four-year-old, a ghost train, and RADA-trained actors dressed as axe-wielding maniacs. We decided against the £12 photographic reminder of the trauma, opting instead to pocket the cash and add it to the savings pot required for future therapy.

Selflessness

Camping. A fate worse than festivals. It's my worst one – my WORST one. If you have to build the accommodation that you're staying in, to me it is not a holiday ... it's a prison job. When the kids came along, my more outdoorsy than me husband took great joy in telling me that now I was a mum I'd have to do 'fun' things like riding a bike and camping. I know some people love it, and I genuinely hope they get the help that they so desperately need, but if I'm peeing in a bush and sleeping on the floor, only to be woken up at 5 a.m. by a bunch of squawking birds, I want it to be because I'm hammered on a hen party. It's just not fun, and I'm very passionate about expressing that – especially if you throw kids into the mix. You're constantly worrying about them running off out of insecure zippy doors; regardless of the time of year, it'll be freezing; and worst of all ... there's always a knobhead with an acoustic guitar somewhere on the campsite. 'Someone's crying, lord ...' ME, I'm crying!

Steve recently bought a six-man tent, thinking that might entice me. Sorry, not even if the six men in question were from *Magic Mike* would I step foot inside that sweaty plastic bag. Of course, you say these things, but then you get emotionally blackmailed by your kids into making 'precious wholesome childhood memories' and so you spend the whole night irrationally scared of a T-rex sticking its head in or a murderer pinpointing your precise location in a Welsh field and killing everyone in their sleep. Of course, that never happens ... because you don't fucking sleep! The whole night is spent desperately needing a phantom wee in a spider-infested toilet 500 metres down a dirt track inspired by a horror movie. My physical, and facial, appearance also rapidly deteriorates by a solid 90 per cent the minute I step foot inside a tent, meaning I leave the whole camping experience not only feeling fifty years older, but looking it too. At least the kids had fun! What's that? They got eaten alive by mosquitoes, traumatised by a badger, and developed frostbite in nineteen of their twenty digits sleeping outside in July? Of course they did.

Resilience

As a parent, your own birthdays are a bit shit, aren't they? Do you know what my kids gave me last year? Conjunctivitis. I did get a 'real' present too … a peg with a pipe cleaner attached to it. When it comes to their birthdays, though, you pull out all the stops. My biggest tradition for the kids is insisting on making their cakes myself. Giving them free rein over Pinterest, every year they always pick the most ludicrous and extremely out of my skill-set fondant-based work of art for me to completely massacre. By the time I've finished making it, four days later and with every kitchen surface covered in icing sugar, it wouldn't look out of place in the dog's dinner bowl. Peppa Pig's head may look like a giant melty cock and balls, but it's been made with love – and that's all that matters … well that and posting it on Instagram for likes. Birthday parties are a logistical nightmare too … guest-list politics, venue sorting, food, entertainment, goody bags. Your kids will also work themselves up into an absolute frenzy about it – on the run-up they'll need to know the exact days, hours, and minutes remaining until their big moment. When party day finally arrives they spend the first hour crying and clinging to your leg as though it's 1912 in the north Atlantic Ocean and you're about to be put on separate lifeboats. It's up to Roy, the overly enthusiastic entertainer who looks as though he should be on a police register, to liven things up with a spot of balloon modelling. Unfortunately, he can only make poodles or phallic-shaped crowns, and both inadvertently end up being used as weapons. There's also nothing quite like the high cortisol feeling of man-marking fifty hyper kids on a bouncy castle, all smacked off their tits on Haribo, to make you think Jehovah's Witnesses have the right idea by not celebrating birthdays. But that's just the calm before the storm. Soon, balloons are going off like grenades and you feel as though you're in a budget remake of *Saving Private Ryan*. And the screaming? Oh, dear God, the screaming – likened only to a cacophony of randy howler monkeys. An hour in … Roy's rocking in a corner, a T-shirtless wild-eyed boy called Tommy has orchestrated a *Lord of the Flies* scenario, and seven Queen Elsas are hysterically sobbing because their eyes have been welded together with glitter tattoos. But it's not time to go yet, no … first there is the ceremonial eating of the party food – where parents arise from the fight-pit circle to stand behind their designated child so they can watch over them like a beige-hunting hawk. 'No party rings for you until you've eaten all of your processed meat!' Finally, the two hours are up. Thank God. Time for party bags, a napkin of cake the birthday child has definitely slobbered on, and to lie down in a very dark room with a very large bottle of alcohol.

Godliness

'Twas the night before Kidmass, when all through the house
a drunk mum was slurring – including her spouse;
The stockings weren't yet hung by the chimney with care,
they'd run out of Sellotape and were shouting a swear;

> The children were nestled all snug in their beds,
> while visions of out-of-stock Nintendos danced in their heads;
> And mama full of anxious grief, and papa who no longer gave two craps,
> accepted their 5 a.m. wake-up with tequila nightcaps …

Christmas! A season my children think is something to do with the birth of baby cheeses, and apparently the most wonderful time of the year. Is it, though? For parents it kind of feels like the most stressful time of the year, especially as your children have been asking how long it is until the big day since the previous year's Boxing Day. There's all the shopping to contend with, social comitments, daily threats … 'I'M GOING TO CALL HIM! DON'T MAKE ME CALL HIM!' And the fear of not procuring the one gift on the list they really want, even though they keep changing their mind, is heightened by a child who has already given their wish list to the Santa who came to school and won't tell anyone else what was on it. The list is obviously essential for a joyous Christmas morning – but more importantly, for leverage. 'If you batter your brother one more time with his own slipper, you can say goodbye to that Lego Frozen castle!' Of course, there's also disciplinary help on hand in the form of the revolutionary 'Santa Cam'. Motion sensors, standby lights on the TV, the green light in your smoke detector – if it's got a bulb, it's perfect for scaring them into submission. I'm not entirely sure how comfortable we should all be with telling our children a fat old man with previous for breaking and entering can see into their homes. A little bit creepy, but effective …

It's also the perfect time of year to be put to shame for not being as fun as all the other mums your child knows. Prime example of this, 'Elf on the Shelf'. Why, why, why would you make life any harder than it already is?! You have children for

Cheesus Christ's sake! The last thing anyone wants to be doing, after crawling into bed at 1 a.m. after too many mulled wines, is setting up a hostage scene between a criminally insane imp and several terrified Disney princess dolls. Just leave him on the sodding shelf, slowly collecting dust along with all your kids' swimming badges and 'star of the week' certificates. He's a bad influence who does not belong in your child's life and should be categorised in the same ASBO bracket as Horrid Henry and Norman Price. Someone bought one for our kids, but weirdly, his hands were stitched to his crotch – causing Evelyn to be very concerned about why he was always holding his winkie. A valid point. I do have a question for the inventors of what I now like to call 'Leprechaun with the Horn', and that is, why do you hate parents so much? I appreciate its origin might have been a cute little family tradition that started when your kids were small, but a vast majority of parents don't have the time or have more important traditions to crack on with – like drinking and over-indulging in pastry. With this in mind, I've created my own new tradition that is much lower maintenance – it's called 'help yourself to one from the top shelf' whereby you pick a bottle of booze, and do a shot. Merry Christmas!

There's all the school social commitments to get involved with too – discos, fairs, raffles, Christmas jumper day, the nativity, party day, toy day, charity shoe box day, own clothes day, paint a bauble, and Christingle … 'Just take all of my pounds and be gone!' Bah! Humbug. The worst of all the activities you have to partake in, however, is the Christmas grotto. A shopping centre, local pub car park, or a hellmouth – regardless of its location, you'll have to queue for two hours in sub-zero temperatures to see the least convincing Santa going, dressed in six metres of Hobbycraft's finest red felt. The worst experience we've ever had of this was the time our friends convinced us to travel an hour and half to a reindeer 'experience' that was supposedly as magical as Lapland itself. Firstly, it was impossible to find – the postcode was null and void, and we ended up in some dodgy-looking business park that looked as though it was more likely to house rats than reindeer. With all the passive aggression, and just plain shouting, we weren't paying attention to Jack in the back asking if he could open the window. Twenty seconds later the whole car was pebble-dashed with a vat of child-vomit. Eventually finding the car park, we tried our hardest to sort out the sick situation – having not thought to bring spare clothes for him, we had to scoop the sick from his now very sad-looking Christmas jumper with our hands, and throw his coat on over the top of him. All the drama meant we'd missed our allotted time slot; our friends had gone ahead without us and we were told to join the painfully long line for the theatre show and grotto. Turns out, the 'magical' experience was one scabby reindeer – potentially a donkey with a branch stuck to its head – standing outside a Portakabin decorated with pound-shop tinsel and empty Foster's cans. Inside wasn't much better – we had to sit through a twenty-minute festive am-dram production while Evelyn complained loudly about a horrible smell (her brother). After queuing up for a further hour, we finally got to meet Santa, who, just finishing off his fag, was located in an extremely seedy red room that looked as though it was normally home to a completely different type of 'lapland'. Perfect. Heading back to the car with two children, who after all of that had been given the gifts of matching pencils, we vowed to NEVER succumb to the peer pressure of grotty grottos EVER again. Until next year, of course …

The key to being a great 'fun mum' is to keep expectation levels at a low baseline, and remember to never peak too soon during long stretches of time, like school holidays. Going too hard, too soon, early doors will only result in feelings of failure in the subsequent weeks as you scream at the TV 'YES,

NETFLIX, WE ARE STILL WATCHING *PEPPA PIG* – YOU JUDGY PIECE OF SHIT.' Most importantly, we can't be expected to be on our entertaining A game at all times of our children's lives – it's impossible and bloody expensive. One thing I know is that the many perfect pictures you see on Instagram have been orchestrated – smoke and mirrors that don't show the behind-the-camera scenes of a mother threatening to take away everything a child has ever loved until they smile nicely, frozen to the bone, in a pumpkin field. So please, don't fall into the trap of comparing yourself and your parenting abilities to others.

If we're being truthful with ourselves, at the end of the day, what actually makes you THE most fun mum is spending one-on-one quality time with your kids. It matters not where that is, and how much money's being spent on them in the process – give them your undivided attention, without a phone in one hand or list of jobs in the other, and they'll be happy as Larry. The only downside is you may have to get the craft box out, or even worse … Junior Monopoly. Regardless, they'll be occupied, and you won't be halfway up Ben Nevis with two children strapped to your back and mountain rescue on speed dial. Cut yourself some slack – the one running through your carabiner, and your psyche.

14

Nature vs Netflix

When you first stare down at that crinkled newborn bundle of pure joy, all snuggly and warm, nestled into your chest as though they're a furless cat in a velour onesie, your heart is filled with such love and adoration you feel it could spontaneously burst into a million pieces at any moment. How is it even possible to love something this much? Their innocence, vulnerability, and complete dependency on you – their creator, their protector, their high priestess. Mummy. It's a love like no other, and one thing's for sure, you can't ever imagine having to utter one cross word at this teeny, tiny, squishy, perfectly perfect human being. There's absolutely no way they'd ever be able to do anything so heinous it'd result in the release of your demented, screechy inner banshee. No. You will be a perfect mother. You'll never raise your voice, implement any kind of punishment, or make any horrid threats. You will be understanding, patient, will listen attentively to all of their stories and problems, believing them wholeheartedly all of the time. Essentially, you'll be a fluffy-slipper-clad version of Ghandi.

If you do experience any slight blips of bad behaviour (unlikely, because this baby has been carved by Angel Gabe himself), you will calmly talk through why their actions have been unacceptable, and of course they'll willingly take on board your constructive criticism – most importantly, learning from it. They'll also love you forever – of course they will, because you are their mother, giver of life, shitter of casseroles, and their best friend ...

Cut to three years later, in the middle of the Tesco dairy aisle, and you've just shouted so loudly at your spawn you've pissed your pants.

'I HATE YOU!'

'I'm sorry ... what did you just say to Mummy?!'

'I HAAAAAAAAAAAAAAAAAAAAAAAAAAAAAAATE YOU!'

'You hate me? The woman whose gut you lived in for nine months, like a chunk of indigestible ribeye? The same lady who endured forty-seven hours of vomit-inducing labour, developed nipples like strawberry laces, and couldn't walk for six weeks after bringing you into the world?'

'Ummmm ...'

'The husk of a once carefree, inny belly-buttoned female who is now unable to leave the house to see her friends without first writing a 150 page instruction manual on how to operate children, and grills?'

'... yes?'

Brilliant.

I'm not *exactly* sure of the precise moment my kids were fed after midnight, but at some point they went from cute and cuddly to slime-covered, Nerf-gun-toting, anarchy-worshipping gremlins. Oh, and did I mention? They are absolutely not my best friends – something my daughter takes great pleasure in informing me of regularly. 'Mummy, you are old and your breath smells. Libby is my best friend.' Harsh.

To be fair, I don't even want them as my BFFs. No, my idea of a bestie is someone who shares my appreciation of explicit Dwayne 'The Rock' Johnson dreams, and is game for smuggling gin miniatures into the school Christmas fair – not someone who continually asks me when I'm going to die, then goes off on one à la John McEnroe because I've given them peas for dinner.

That moment when a child you love so unequivocally that you'd be willing to sacrifice your own life … partner for enthusiastically and zealously expresses their hatred for you is absolutely horrific. Cuts like a blunt Thomas the Tank Engine knife through your heart as they venomously spit out the words, all while smashing your face in with a lightsaber. It's the look in their eyes too, when they say it … they really mean it. It's as though the contempt's been building up inside them for a while, very similar to my husband's feelings for me during the Great Lockdown of 2020 when he was only one god-awful period fart away from a manslaughter plea.

It's an emotional blow that'll no doubt compound your feelings of being the world's worst parent, all because you refused to let them stick a fork in a toaster or lick an open flame. MONSTER. I cried the first time my son said it. Steve, who has a stronger grasp on reason than I do, tried to talk me down from the 'do we need a child psychologist?' ledge. 'Babe, don't take it personally. It's just what kids say when they don't know how to properly express their feelings.' It felt pretty personal as I was having my face rearranged with the full power of the force.

I feel pa*renting* is somewhat the wrong term to describe the daily carnage of childrearing. It provides you with an almost misleading assumption that it's a casual arrangement – something that potentially holds a break clause after six months, allowing you to just pack up and fuck off somewhere more exciting. This is not the case. Par*owning*, I feel, is a much fairer representation of the situation – financially crippling and ties you in for at least thirty-five years. It's a tough gig. It's even more difficult trying to teach your kid how to be a decent person, when you're not entirely sure your own moral fibre is up to muster …

But it's all so romantic, isn't it, planning that first baby – what flavour it'll be, the hopes and dreams for their future, who it'll resemble? You, your other half, or that weird cousin in the family who looks like they've dabbled with meth? You don't really put much thought into 'how' they're going to turn out and the part you'll play in crafting that persona. Will it be down to nature, or Netflix? One thing I do know is that once you've finally emerged from those 'cute' yet exhausting baby years, you're going to be left with a very real, not always as endearing human being that you're responsible for dragging up and teaching to be a respectable, valued member of society. The only real measure of your success will be if you can get them to 21 and they're not in jail, or still sleeping in your bed. The journey will be fun, though – lots of grunting, experimenting with drink, drugs, and a whole load of bad life choices. Same goes for the kids too. Anyway, there's a part of me that thinks you don't actually become a 'parent' until you've had to explain why siblings aren't allowed to touch each other's private parts. 'YOU JUST CAN'T!' Anything up until that point is just a basic carer's role of feeding them, turning on the kids' channel, and not letting the dog lick them directly in the mouth.

I'm thinking that maybe a couple of top-up modules on crime and punishment should be added on to antenatal classes for extra parenting credit? Effective techniques on how to deal with screamers, spitters, and sass pots, because there's still so much I don't really know how to deal with. My current parenting modus operandi for dealing with my kids' antics is to pretend I'm calling the fuzz on them – 'Hello, is this Officer Dibble? Oh, I'm afraid there's been a serious case of ABH. Yes, that's right, Arguing, Biting, Hitting …' – then having to live with the fear of knowing 'snitches get stitches'.

One of my biggest anxieties, aside from being shivved with a filed-down Minions toothbrush, is that I'll handle a parenting situation so badly my kids will grow up to be throat-slashing serial killers – or worse, traffic wardens. I wonder whether mothers of prolific monsters lie awake at night wondering where it all went horribly wrong. Was it because they'd forgotten they'd put them on the naughty step, only realising three hours later when Netflix questioned 'Are you *still* watching *Tiger King*?' Maybe, back in the eighteenth century, Jack the Ripper's mummy took away his Apple products for six years too? 'No more Pink Ladies for you, young man!' Leaving him to think 'I'll show you …'

I'll admit, I have no idea how to correctly parent my occasionally 'spirited' kids (which is Waitrose for 'naughty'), not even the second born – which you'd think would be easier because I've already been through terrorist negotiation training with the first. But it's not. Somehow it's more difficult because they hunt together, reminiscent of a pair of *Jurassic Park* velociraptors, working together in tandem to pin me down.

Essentially, it's my own fault that I'm now outnumbered by smarter genetic adaptations of my own DNA who have not only learnt to open the sharp knife drawer, but can also recite the passcodes to every electronic device they've ever encountered. I grew up with an older sister so was very much on board with the creation of a fellow playmate, but having spent the past four years refereeing the sibling spin-off of *Fight Club*, occasionally there are days when I question the logic behind that idea … Yes, there are moments of pure, unadulterated, harmonious joy, when they play together so sweetly I feel as though my life choices have been 100 per cent affirmed. Then, there are days when one has the other in a chokehold and I've screamed so loudly the neighbours have knocked on to see if we're all OK.

I'll call out the biggest myth about par*owning*. Listening ears! What a crock of shit. How do I get them? Are they in-ear purchases I have to pay extra for? I hear teachers and other parents talking about them, but my kids don't seem to have access to them yet. Listening ears, kind hands, gentle mouths – utter bollocks! I demand to know who pretend-invented these terms so I can find their home address and swear at them with my unkind mouth to stop making body parts into Good Samaritans – it's not a real thing! I was absolutely convinced my children had actual hearing problems, only to discover they were just choosing to ignore me. Parents in a similar predicament, let me save you the worry – just go into a different room from your kids, open a pack of biscuits and put something you want to watch on the TV – if within three seconds they're on you like flies on shit, they're fine.

My kids seem to live their lives by the strangely worrying youth culture of 'YOLO' – You Only Listen Once, when you're about twelve months old … to your own name – after that, no more information is required. I worry I've potentially lost my fear factor with them – they've been so overexposed to my primal roaring it now just washes over them like white noise. I'm essentially a Spotify playlist: 'Mummy's relaxing jungle sounds'. At one point over the summer holidays, I decided to conduct a social experiment to see what would happen if I gave up yelling for twenty-four hours. My voice had nothing to lose and my pelvic floor had everything to gain. Instead, I opted to embody the cool, calm and collected Liam Neeson in *Taken*. It worked for about five minutes, then my son assumed I was drunk or medicated and so decided to take advantage by proceeding to beat the crap out of his little sister – all while I attempted to convince him I'd acquired a very particular set of skills that'd make his life a living nightmare.

'If you let my daughter go now, that'll be the end of it. Are we using our kind hands?'

'No, I'm using a plastic shovel ...'

Fair enough. Where do you even go from there?

Manners are another combustion point in our household. Cost nothing, do they? My own parents' words coming back to haunt me ... Generally speaking, my kids are good ... in public. Take them out for dinner or to someone's house and they're the most polite children in the universe, which I can't complain about. But at home, with me, I spend hours loudly emphasising 'P-L-E-A-S-E!' after every demand for sustenance, channel-changing, or bum-wiping. DRIVES ME MAD. I've got to the point where I literally refuse to do anything unless it's been requested politely. Steve has also taken note of this for all his after-hours asks ...

Bedtime – a constant struggle. It's the time they dick around the most, and the pressure of trying to convince a child to just go the fuck to sleep is generally always intensified by the fact you've stupidly asked, 'Are you tired?' Wow. Just stand back and watch the transformation from cute, eye-rubbing small human to a slightly less endearing miniature Hulk 'I'M ... NOT ... TIRED!'

A truly terrifying encounter, you need to be prepared for them to come at you aggressively wielding a pair of plastic Crayola scissors and a Frube. 'Bitch, what did you say to me?!' Valuing your eyesight, and foolish choice of a dry clean only jumper, you have to massively backpedal and pretend it just didn't happen. 'Mummy said NOTHING, sweetheart ...'

Why *do* they get so irate about that one question? It's almost as though if they admit defeat just once, the whole jig is then up and they'll be kicked out of their pre-school posse for snitching. I'm telling you, kid cliques are on a par with violent prison gangs – after all, Orange Is the New Blackcurrant …

I've never understood over-tiredness in children. If you're an adult, you sit down, fall asleep and spill a glass of red wine over yourself. For kids, they weirdly acquire more energy, insist on partying as though they're at an illegal rave, then break down in a heap of snot and hysterics. By the same logic, why is over-awake not a thing?

Yes, bedtime for me is a very mixed bag of emotions. It is the best of times; it is the worst of times. A two-hour battle of wills that starts with effectively trying to herd cats up a flight of stairs, bathe them (we all know how much cats love water) and wrangle their bedraggled bodies into pyjamas (or whatever the hell they want to wear, normally a Christmas jumper in July). Someone always gets assaulted by a torch, a toothbrush ends up in the toilet, Daddy comes and shouts for bit, and Mummy threatens to call Father Christmas (again, in July – it's never too early), then there's a suspiciously timed stomach ache/head ache/finger ache/tongue ache, for which enough Calpol is slung down throats for it to be considered a gateway drug, everyone's hungry/thirsty, something's ALWAYS itchy, and guaranteed there'll tears before bed – normally mine. I know people who have their kids in bed and asleep by 7 p.m. I can only assume they've drugged them.

Why don't my kids get tired?! I've tried everything – aside from chloroform (I'm at the stage now where if it was available on Amazon Prime, I'd be tempted). The perfect-parent brigade who have their equally perfect kids in bed early are always the ones who say really helpful things, such as 'Have you tried getting them into a routine?' We have one thanks, that we stick to religiously. I shout at them to go to sleep, they mess around until 10 p.m. asking for crackers, and I listen to a cacophony of

'MUMMY!' wails while singing the *Paw Patrol* theme tune through a closed door.

People say you 'get the child you deserve', which is a lovely sentiment when they're behaving, but for the days you're on the receiving end of a kid who's been given the wrong-coloured plate, you begin to wonder what the hell you did in a past life. I'm sorry, OK? The purple plate's in the dishwasher, Don Fussy Fucker. You're there at bedtime, nervously pulling back the bedding, half expecting to find the severed head of a pink hobby horse on your pillow – a warning shot from the melamine mafia. Why are they so particular about tableware? My daughter once booted off so dramatically over the picking up of a spoon, we have to refer to it as the birth of the Cutlery Utensils Negotiation Treaty due to the extreme length of the arbitration that followed. BREXIT had nothing on it. You see, this wasn't just any old spoon. It was a partially dishwasher-melted orange IKEA plastic spoon. What's wrong with that, you may ask? EVERYTHING to a child who's woken up wanting the PINK Salvador Dali-esque spoon but is relying solely on the power of telepathy and fairies to relay the information. You just can't rationalise with that level of cray, but that doesn't stop you trying – and that, right there, is your first mistake. NEVER negotiate with terrorists. Now, when attempting to bend a child to your will, there is a standard eight-point plan most parents will try to follow. It's a tried and tested blueprint that starts with their least attentive, and our favourite, body part – that's right, those waxy, highly selective lug holes. So, in my best sing-song voice, and mustering all the enthusiasm and exuberance of Snow White after a few lines of coke (Snow by name, snow by nature), I stupidly asked …

'Sweetheart, are we using our listening ears? Pick up the spoon!'

Of course she wasn't. Time to move on to your secret weapon: flattery – notoriously something that gets you everywhere unless, that is, the person you're sweet-talking is three.

'I think somebody here is the best gosh-darn spoon picker-upper in the room!'

She was like, 'Yeah, you. Dickhead. You're the best spoon picker-upper in the room. Just do it already so we can all get on with our day.'

Sensing this was not going quite to the 'Mumsnet Forum' plan, I slid, with the stealth and ease of Neeson, on to the deployment of Phase Three: reverse psychology …

'Oh, I don't think somebody here *can* pick up the spoon. It's just far too difficult …'

This also failed because she just assumed the dextrously challenged idiot in the room was me …

'Come on, Mummy, you can do it! Pretend it's a Jaffa Cake!'

Making a mental note to lay off the biscuits, it was clear things needed to be swiftly escalated to Phase Four: a bit of good old-fashioned good cop, bad cop. Enter 'Player Two' … Daddy.

'Daddy is very cross. Pick up the spoon!'

She was very quick to call bullshit on this. She's seen Daddy very cross from that time Mummy didn't use her 'looking eyes' and scraped half the car off on the gate post. If his neck vein ain't popping, he's just pretending.

Anticipating that victory may already be in the hands of the enemy, it was time for Steve to roll out the fifth element of the campaign – more commonly known as 'Shouty Phase' …

'PICK UP THE SPOON, PICK UP THE SPOON, PICK UP THE SPOON!!!'

Always a gamble, and likely to get you nowhere. By the time Daddy's jugular was doing the samba, she was planning on picking that spoon up at about quarter past NEVER, and having completely lost sight of the original goal, I was right there with her. 'Yeah, babe, that's right – down with the patriarchy!'

After a brief yet heated discussion in the downstairs loo about undermining authority, Mummy and Daddy were ready to bring about Phase Six, the big guns, the AK47s of the parenting world, and more powerful than my Dwayne's biceps – that's right … counting to three in ascending order! Why do we think this will terrify small children into submission? We never learn that steamrolling in there like a draconian Carol Vorderman only leads to two things: a) Genghis Khan't count is unable to do the maths on what comes next after two and three quarters, and b) they know that after 'three' you've got absolutely nothing. The world does not explode in a fiery ball of lava and wrath, and Officer Dibble and his SWAT team do not abseil down from the ceiling to whisk them away to Azkaban. No, fuck all happens.

Now what? Phase Seven: the naughty step. That's all you have left. The fear of sitting still for five minutes, on carpet, while you go and pick up the bastard spoon because you can't cope with having to get to the next part of the programme – the TV ban. At that point, you're only punishing yourselves.

The final step of the process is to extract an apology, under duress, from a child who's spent a fun-filled ten minutes on the stairs playing 'slides' and using your car keys to etch stickmen into the skirting boards.

'Are you sorry?'

'No.'

'ARE YOU SORRY?'

'… Yes?'

'Do you mean that?'

'No.'

'Do you know why Mummy sent you to the naughty step?'

'No …'

'Because you wouldn't pick up the spoon.'

'But Mummy ...'

'WHAT?!'

'... You didn't say please!'

FUCK.

It's all about actions and consequences, people, actions and consequences ...

A lot of the time, I worry horribly about being too hard on the kids ... I just want them to grow up being the best they can be, but am so fearful it's going to be at the detriment of our own relationship. After a heavy day of shouting, empty threats and, of course, rewarding their bad behaviour, I'll lie awake all night torturing myself with how I've handled certain situations, promising that tomorrow I'll do better, be better and, in turn, make them better. Have you ever heard your own stern words come out of your child's mouth while they're playing, their face contorted with faux anger as they boss about a sibling or friend? It's awful. I want so much to be a fun mum all the time – but I also don't want them to get run over, hurt people, set fire to animals, or leave cutlery on the floor. Why is there no straightforward guide on how to tread these perilous parenting planks? Probably because no child is straightforward, or perfect – as much as we may want them to be. And why should they be? I'm not, so why are my expectations of people with a tenth (someone may need to check the maths on that) of my life experience so high?

Yes, there are times we feel as though our kids have walked, no, wait – trampled – all over us, but it's easy to forget they're just little, doing what they do best – laughing, exploring, living, and pushing you towards an early grave. They'll learn, you'll learn, they'll say they hate you and you'll always cry. Of course we also have tons of brilliant days too which make my heart sing with joy, like when Jack and I sit for hours making comics together – he's so talented, creative and funny I could implode with love-filled pride over the little boy I made. Parents and kids won't always be best friends, probably nowhere near – but I know I'll always love them with every fibre of my very being because I'm their Mummy, and what better trump card to have when they're questioning my authority than 'BECAUSE YOU LIVED IN ME!'

15

The Muffia

There comes a devastating point in your parenting career when you'll turn into the proud, yet emotionally unstable, owner of a school-age child. What happened? Where did that time go? The past four to five years have cruelly flown by and it seems so unfair. How did you get to be so bloody old?! They are babies and absolutely not ready to be integrated into the education system, wear little ties, or experience the cut-throat world of primary-school playground thug life. You want to keep them small, covered in bubble wrap and firmly in your sights forever. Will they make new friends? Will you? Will they drink enough? While they're out at school, will you drink too much? WHO WILL WIPE THEIR ARSE?! You are not ready for this in the slightest. Maybe homeschooling is the way forward … your patient and Mother Earth approach to parenting thus far would stand you in good stead, would it not …? Your child, on the other hand, more than likely can't wait to cut the neurotic apron strings and will be chomping at the bit for change. It's not about them, though

... it's about you, and moving onto that next chapter – one predominantly featuring phonetically sounded out words, and if you're very lucky, three twatty kids called Biff, Chip, and Kipper.

Before arriving at primary school, your precious offspring have probably been in some form of formal childcare setting first – nursery, preschool, a playpen with the iPad, etc. School, however, feels like a completely different ball game. It's the start of their journey into adulthood – the decisions you make now could have massive ramifications on their future. It's not like choosing a nursery, where you judge it on smell and how much crusty green snot you can see on an 18-month-old baby. Picking the wrong school could shape their friendship group, educational progression, and chances of developing ... intestinal worms. When it came to deciding on where Jack was going, I did as all good, caring, and educationally well-informed mothers do ... and selected the one closest to my house. But wait, what's that? Just because you've picked a school doesn't mean you automatically get in. No, annoyingly, there's a whole process involving geographical location, sibling priorities, religious beliefs, emotional blackmail, and an openness to bribery. Our chosen school, 0.1 miles away from our front door, just so happened to be Church of England affiliated. Now, I'm not 'not' religious, I just happen to have a few teeny tiny unanswered questions on some of the finer details ... dinosaurs, evolution, two people getting jiggy and populating the whole world, etc. – all of which I was willing to sweep under the carpet in the name of an extra ten minutes in bed and a swifter school run. Despite our proximity to our desired school, the only guaranteed way of securing a place was a signed letter from the local vicar verifying our involvement in the religious community. So close, so far. In the same way God's ultimate sacrifice was sending his only son to earth to die, mine was sending myself to church, hungover, every Sunday to do the same. I swear the holy water bubbled every time we took our seats (late) at the back, our children's booming voices vocalising their need for a poo during silent prayer times, and me desperately trying to hush Evelyn every time she excitedly pointed out the 'Butterfly man!'

'No, sweetheart, that's Jesus ... on the cross.' Also worth pointing out, a sip of communion wine filled with the saliva of sixty parishioners is not ideal the morning after eight margaritas. 'The blood of Christ?'

'Any chance of a Diet Coke?'

Waiting for confirmation of that first primary-school place is properly nervewracking. In a strategic approach, I purposefully chose two backup schools we were very unlikely to be given – one being oversubscribed, the other being in Belarus. There might have also been a bullshit *War and Peace*-length essay sent to the local education authority about our efforts to be a 'foot-powered', carbon-neutral family with a clinically obese dog ... Whether it was location, luck, or with a bit of help from the big man ('Six-Foot-Sam at the council), we were in!

The first time your child dons their school uniform, all dressed up like they belong in an 'Employee of the Month' hall of fame, needs to come with a mental health warning. It's just too goddamn much. Granted, they need to grow up – can't stay little forever, like Hobbits – but you're also so worried about letting them go off into the big wide world on their own. Who's going to check their breathing every twenty minutes? WHAT IF THERE'S AN UNCUT GRAPE?! It's such a big change for everyone, and I don't like change. Steve once bought me supermarket own-label tampons and I cried – completely irrational, but also valid because it wasn't just my eyes that leaked.

Having spent the entirety of the summer trying to teach your kid how to wipe their own arse, 'FRONT TO BACK!', the big day is finally upon you. First, there's the token front-door picture for Instagram, before heading off on the school run – a painfully slow funeral march … towards the death of your youth. Entering the playground, hundreds of seemingly gigantic screeching children bustle past you, twatting each other with water bottles and shooting one another with stick guns. Holding onto your angelic baby for dear life, you're never letting go and most certainly are not leaving them alone at HMP (Her Majesty's Primary) 'Eye Poke'. If push comes to shove, you're going in with them. Still unable to recite the nine times table, repeating early years education seems to be a practical solution to a combination of crippling overbearingness, and slight numerical dyslexia.

Arriving at the building, there's wailing, a reluctance to leave, and someone's just had an anxiety wee on the hopscotch – it's reassuring to know fellow parents are also taking it as badly. The children, however – absolutely fine. Zero fucks given. They've already made friends and are licking one another. Suddenly, the doors open and reception teachers swoop into the nervous crowd like ravenous birds of prey, plucking kids from the arms of hysterical parents and hurling them into classrooms faster than a Venus Williams serve. Your babies don't even glance back as the doors slam shut behind them. Absolutely brutal. Sobbing mothers are littered all over the playground, makeshift triages have been set up for those on the ground being comforted by random strangers. 'They'll be OK, babe, you've got this!' Others are lashing out at eye-rolling dads who are unhelpfully reminding them they'll be back in two hours to collect them. Tearstained, you arrive home. The house feels strange, empty, and quiet. It dawns on you, you're either totally on your own, or a child down and it's … MARVELLOUS! It's actually amazing how quickly you get over them starting school once you realise you can have a wee without somebody constantly criticising the state of your bush.

Something that becomes apparent in your new role as a school mum is that you are much more likely to get the American government to spill their guts on Area 51 than you are to get your kids to share details of their highly secretive day. It would appear that on entering the education system, they are required to sign a non-disclosure agreement prohibiting the sharing of any information about what they've done, who they've played with, or whether they've had a jacket potato for lunch. You ponder whether instead of reading and writing, they're actually at spy school being taught anti-interrogation techniques.

'What did you do today, sweetheart?'

'I don't remember …' You've literally just greeted them at the threshold of the classroom door.

'How can you not remember something that happened thirty seconds ago?!' You realise that, coming from you, there's a certain amount of irony in that statement.

'Well, what did you have for lunch?' From the state of their face and jumper, it was beans, with a side of yogurt – but you want to hear it from the horse's crusty-looking mouth.

'I DON'T REMEMBER!'

Right, that's that then. No amount of trickery or bribery can break them. They offer a solidarity nod towards their teacher that says 'I didn't say a fucking word, guv' before turning their attention to quizzing you … 'Mummy, did you bring a snack?' While they're patting you down for a KitKat, as though you might be harbouring a weapon or sharps, there's time to assess the only evidence pointing away from a day's worth of firearms training – an empty Colgate box with a pipe cleaner glued to it. That's right, SHART. This is especially prevalent in Reception – a million trees give their lives annually in order for you to be joyfully presented with a poster-paint interpretation of a murder scene. I guarantee, most parents of school-age children will have at one point or another uttered these exact words 'Oh, it's brilliant, darling! What is it?' I imagine little Pablo Picasso's mum didn't go home with a Lidl Multigrain Hoops box covered in feathers and file it under 'recycling'. And the portraits are even more terrifying. Halfway through Jack's first year, I seriously had to reconsider my go-to staple hairstyle of the 'mum bun' after a series of unfortunate pictures came home of me seeming to have a gigantic cock on my head …

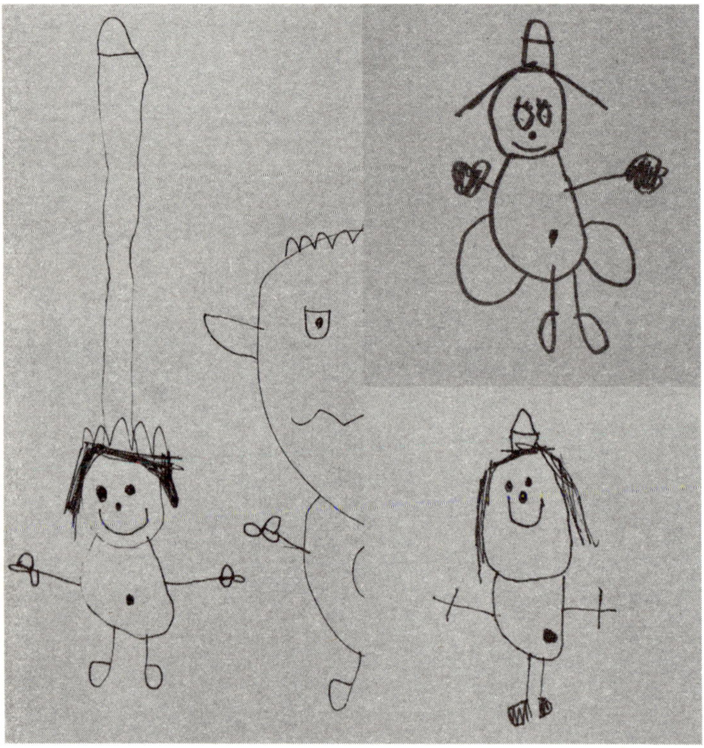

Could have been worse, there could have been a picture of Steve flying a helicopter with his 'chopper' out … oh wait …

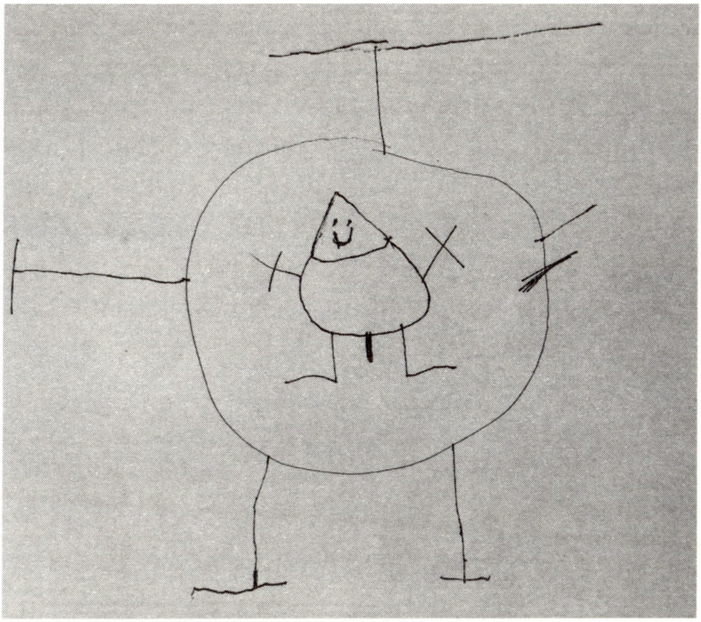

With school life comes the worry of falling in with the wrong crowd, and of course gang culture … Ross Kemp ain't seen NOTHING until he's stepped foot inside a primary school and witnessed, first-hand, the dark underbelly of … suburban mum-life. Which crew you belong to depends on several contributing factors. Are you, for example, part of the Gossip Gang? A highly dangerous clique who like to menacingly loiter at the gates, ready to pounce on the most meagre of hearsay and permeate it through all year groups via a vast network of informants. Or, are you more of a Drop and Ditch Bitch? No interest in playground niceties – get in, chuck you kid through a door, get out. Streamlined and efficient, they care not about meaningless conversations surrounding the weather, PE kit politics, especially don't give a shit about anyone's plans for the weekends, and would rather cut out their own tongue than help at the school fair. Then there's the New Baby Buddies, with their turf centred mainly around a local Costa Coffee – no one's slept in six months, everything hurts and leaks, plus they've accidentally come out in slippers. They do, however, have the best wheels on the playground – a Bugaboo deluxe travel system. If you're highly organised, are a parent representative, and never forget the forest school kit, you're more than likely in the Smug Squad. At the helm of collecting money for staff Christmas presents (always a bottle of Prosecco and framed sentimental tat that'll be left in a classroom drawer), their shit is firmly held together, and fingers are constantly on the pulse when it comes every aspect of school life – fairs, bake sales, who's not paid their lunch money on the parent app. Membership into this highly prestigious group is not without its risks, nor is it permanent ... the minute you get curly-fingered by a teacher because your kid assaulted another child with Duplo, you're out and forced into the dreaded no-mum's land.

Then there's my own special kind of people ... the Punctually Impaired Posse, or PIPs for short. Disorganised, dishevelled, and done in – no matter what time we wake or how early we leave the house, we will always be legging it through those gates with sweat dripping off our chins, barking orders at our lacking-in-urgency offspring to hurry the fuck up, and looking like we've been roughed up by an aggressive squirrel. Last but not least, and responsible for keeping us all in check, is the most terrifying group of them all ... The Muffia, otherwise known as the PTA (Playground Territorial Army). Formed from a formidable network of overly enthusiastic parents, they are a force to be reckoned with. Not so much of a choice, but a calling. You don't mess with the mum mob – when they WhatsApp, you answer. Never try to feign illness, or make up an awful excuse because resistance is futile – come 5 December, you both know who's going to be at the Christmas fete manning the bastard teddy tombola.

Something that unites all us mamas, though, is our choice of uniform – and I don't mean grey pinafores and easy-iron shirts (which for the record: not easy). Ask yourself this question, and answer honestly … Are you even a school mum if you haven't done the school run dressed in any of these items?

1. *Bobble hat.* A necessity for any knackered, greasy-haired mum on a cold morning. Faux-fur rabbit's arse on the top is a fashion MUST. Why waste precious dry shampoo when you can hide your shit hair under this winter playground essential? Come summertime, either replace with a baseball cap, or actually wash your hair. Needs must.
2. *Padded coat, furry hood.* If you can't survive in −18°C arctic conditions while walking to school in June, then you ain't on trend. With a furry hood that'd give Tina Turner's hair a run for its money, this half woman, half lion look is perfect for rainy days, the transferal of head lice, and getting yourself run over due to a dramatically reduced peripheral vision. Big pockets are essential for easy storage of half-eaten cereal bars, crumb-coated raisins, a few bus tickets from three years ago, and the possible root cause of Covid. Can be worn with, or without, big patches of mud up the front and back from picking up children who can't be arsed to walk.
3. *Activewear.* A must-have staple in any self-respecting school-run-mum's wardrobe. These elasticated, high waisted Lycra lovelies are comfortable, practical and, unlike their evil cousin the skinny jean, don't induce IBS. They may have banned pyjamas in the playground, but naff-all has been said about leggings. Wear at bedtime, then get up and rock a look that sticks two fingers up to the

establishment. Rebel. Crucially, when wearing them, it is of the utmost importance you are not active. Biscuits are a yes, burpees are a no.

4. *Ugg Boots.* These glorified slippers keep toes toasty, while their thick tread makes it near impossible to completely remove all traces of dog shit from them. Swap to Converse in the summer months for an 'I'm still down with the kids' hipster vibe. Especially 'en vogue' when worn with your in-activewear.
5. *Scooter.* This two/three-wheeled contraption of death is to be worn casually draped over the shoulder, and can be accessorized with a child who is refusing to use it. Finish off the look with a plaster cast, from when you tried to scoot home from school but fell into a bush.
6. *Dog. Optional.* Nothing says 'multi-tasking the shit out of life' better than a dog with explosive bowels and separation anxiety. This fluffy object can either be handheld, attached to a pram – dragging the wearer down the road and into the path of oncoming traffic – or tied to a gate in order to bark at small children and old people. The dog is a brave, and acquired, choice – not for the fashion faint-hearted – or Ugg boot-wearer.

As the official spokesperson of the PIPs, it probably comes as no surprise that I find the school run possibly one of the most challenging elements of school life. Before embarking on the journey of motherhood, no one told me it'd be easier to get a child out of your body than it would be to get them out of the house in the morning. SO much dicking around. Firstly, no one wants to get out of bed – probably something to do with staying up all night shouting for crackers and Calpol. Embodying the spiritual essence of a pre-menstrual ogre, you surprise even yourself at the furious guttural roar you're able to emit from your body pre-8 a.m. It takes so long arguing about the necessity of a morning wee, discussing the meaning of life, and manipulating non-compliant arms into dresses, jumpers and shirts, etc., there's no time to make yourself look presentable. Yet again, you'll be jogging up to school looking like you've had a heavy night on the crack. At breakfast, tensions rise even further, especially if you have more than one child you're trying to get out of the door at the same time. Your eldest kid has got to the cereal cupboard first and has managed to consume the last of the Cheerios, leaving the youngest with a fate worse than cornflakes … Weetabix. It's kicking off like a football derby day – chokeholds, tear gas, and horses (hobby, used as weapons).

As someone who is habitually disorganised, I pride myself on never having the foresight to prepare the lunchboxes the night before. Would it make my life 50 per cent easier in the mornings? Absolutely. Am I ever going to learn from my mistakes? Never. While the kids are upstairs, best friends again, squealing with laughter and NOT brushing their teeth as requested upwards of eight times, it's time to scour the bare cupboards in an attempt to provide something vaguely acceptable to children who'll only eat food in stick form. Cheese Strings, Peperamis, Choobs (like Frubes but a quid cheaper) and a slightly flattened banana all get lobbed in while you pray the 'midday assistants' (posh for 'dinner ladies') don't closely inspect the high-sugar, high-salt excuse for nutrition you've bunged in. Teeth still haven't been brushed, no one can find any shoes, a kid has decided to go for a twenty-minute poo, and your heart rate has peaked as though you're midway through a spin class.

'FACES! COATS! DRINKS BOTTLE! LUNCH BOX! SHOES ON RIGHT FEET! STOP PLAYING WITH LEGO! I DON'T

KNOW WHY FROGS CAN BREATHE UNDER WATER AND ON LAND. LET'S GO!'

On your marks, get set … drag! Thirty minutes later (it should take ten), with blood pressure through the roof and ankles shredded from the bastard stunt scooter, you arrive at the gates with one minute to spare. Hurrah, victory! Celebrating with a fist punch to the air, you suddenly notice every other child apart from your own … is dressed like a pirate. FUCK'S SAKE! International Talk Like a Pirate Day. Not even a proper thing! But there you are, regardless, stood in the middle of the playground trying to fashion an eyepatch out of a sanitary towel and digging a euro out of your purse. 'Just chuck it in the pot, it looks the same – no one will know.'

You will have never noticed the similarities between your child and an Asda shopping trolley until they start school – can't go anywhere without a quid. It's never-ending – own clothes day, Children in Need, Comic Relief, Sports Relief, decorate a mythical creature day, crazy hair day, a fundraiser for the local aardvark sanctuary, paint a cardboard box day/the teacher's Christmas party fund. How are we meant to remember them all?! Granted, I could actually read the newsletter, or unmute the WhatsApp groups, but that would result in me having to trawl through hundreds of daft questions like 'If it's snowing, can we send them in with gloves?' No. Teachers would much prefer them to develop frostbite so their fingers fall off – stops them picking their dirty little noses. My personal favourite of all the days is World Book Day. If you think those PRICKs were bad when their kids were little, you're in for a treat when their prodigies hit school age and there's an opportunity to combine a love of literature with an industrial glue gun. It's not about their child, who wants to go dressed as a superhero from their favourite book – the Argos catalogue. No, it's actually an opportunity for Twats R Us to showcase their replica Hogwarts headdress, made out of 6000 toilet roll holders and layers of fingertip skin. For all disorganised parents, there's nothing quite like the panic realisation of discovering there's not enough time to Amazon Prime something to yourself, resulting in a mad dash around Hobbycraft and purchasing enough spray paint to raise suspicions of Banksy's identity. An all-nighter later, off your tits on aerosol fumes, you have a child's outfit that wouldn't look out of place on the SHART shelf. Instead of books, one year our school decided to do a 'Vocabulary Parade'. Being an uninformed shit parent who had no idea what the hell that was, twenty-four hours prior to said event Google told me it was just another opportunity for parents to swing their massive dic … tionaries. Instead of going as their favourite literary classic, children dress as their favourite word – which, to be frank, is a terrible idea because show me a seven-year-old whose favourite word isn't 'bum', and I'll show you a liar. When his classmates were going as Pinterest-worthy 'precipitation', or 'foliage', I could hardly dress the kid as a gigantic arse hole, despite him occasionally acting like one.

As well as watching out for pound-depleting days, you'll constantly need your wits about you so as not to fall prey to the worst fate a primary school parent can face … volunteering. Volunteering?! Sorry, you want me to help you look after my kid? There must be a mistake … I've done that for four years already – they're all yours now, aren't they?! I was planning on having a midday wine and watching thirty-two back-to-back episodes of *Come Dine with Me*. Unfortunately, danger lurks everywhere … school trips, laminating, cutting and sticking, LISTENING TO KIDS READ! The worst one by far. Honestly, I used to think of myself as a good, kind, caring mother … up until the point I was introduced to phonics.

'D-O-G'

'Well done, sweetheart, so what's the word?'

'Cat!'

'We've been reading a story about Floppy the dog for an hour now, darling. There's a big fuck-off golden retriever on every page, so no – not cat!'

There was a particularly dark moment in my life, when 'Bob Bug' was sent home in the book bag, or as my child insisted on calling him … Bill.

'No darling, l-i-s-t-e-n. *Every* page starts with the word 'Bob', OK? Got it?'

'Yes, Mummy!'

'Lovely, let's try again, shall we?'

'Bill bug …'

There's now a small, six-legged creepy-crawly-shaped hole in my soul that will never be repaired. A word of warning – when teaching small people how to read, never forget the addition of gin to your phonics.

World Book Day, sadly, will not be the only time you'll encounter a PRICK. At every step of your child's schooling life, there they'll be, boasting about their special sperm's 'lead' in the Christmas nativity (sheep number one), how brilliant they are at sports (is throwing other kids into brick walls considered an Olympic sport?), and, of course, their natural academic prowess … 'Little Edward's so advanced, you know … he's been doing quantum physics since he was three.'

You don't get involved because your kid, like most of their age group, is still writing their name backwards, and last week asked if chipmunks were made out of chips. No, Kcaj, they are not. Edward might very well be a genius, but here's a question … can he put his own shoes on? Seems to be an ability that eludes ALL children, regardless of intellect, until circa 17. Little Einstein may be on Gold Band reading books but give him a Clarks light-up dinosaur shoe and it'll be like his hands have been replaced with shovels.

The best time, however, to observe the PRICKs in their natural habitat is on Sports Day – the most highly competitive day in the calendar, again, not for the children. Training for this monumental event will have started months in advance, despite women in Nike Lycra two-pieces claiming they haven't done any cardio for months – this is total bullshit. They've been pounding the pavements harder than Sir Mo Farah. On the start line, the tension is palpable ... the kids are cheering, the dads are filming, the mums are jostling for prime position – many of the under-prepared and emotionally blackmailed are holding onto their boobs for dear life. 'On your marks, get set ... fucking leg it!' It's an eventful race, with Tina from Year 2 taking an early lead, only to be robbed, in the dying seconds, by a Reception mum in a pair of Yeezys who victoriously celebrates with a 'mumbot'. Tina, absolutely seething and furiously demanding to see the VAR, has to be removed from the premises by security (Mr Jones, the caretaker). The dads' race is just as eventful; however, there's no need for a photo finish as half have fallen arse over man-tit within two feet of the start, and the rest are crawling their way to the finish line with ruptured hamstrings. It's a war scene – wet paper towels and cold compresses everywhere. Eventually the prize is awarded to the bloke with the most remaining, fully intact limbs.

Yes, your children starting school can be a terrifying prospect for all, but not as terrifying, however, as the moment you discover they've illegally smuggled a host of new pets home with them ... in their hair. HEAD LICE! Levelling with you, they are my worst fear (camping aside). I did not sign up for that shit when I committed to motherhood. A whole ecosystem thriving on their bonces – reproducing, building infrastructure, shagging like mad, outsmarting modern science – and you don't notice them until they're big enough to leave home and fly the nest ... onto your own head. Cruelly, by the time you make the grim discovery, they've already infiltrated your entire household through towels, bedding, hairbrushes, and of course patient X, who just *loves* snuggling up to you at night. It's all kicking off on the WhatsApp group too – no one knows which child has spread it, but speculation is rife, with the infestation causing a raging war of words between rival gang members and parents 'leaving' the groups in an indignant rage. The day prior to their detection in our household, we'd had a birthday party for Evelyn – tens of little girls, all with beautiful long, flowing locks, happily frolicking around on a bouncy castle together. Sending the bad-news WhatsApp message less than twenty-four hours later could, I imagine, rival the shame of getting in touch with past partners to tell them you've got chlamydia. 'Thanks so much for coming yesterday! Hope you all enjoyed your cake and blood-leaching hair parasites!' Worst fucking goodie bag EVER. I wasn't prepared for them in the slightest – having had a boy first, I'd managed to get seven years into parenting without ever running into one of the fuckers. Going to hold my hands up here and say I *possibly* didn't handle it all that well … er, I might have screamed in my child's face. In my defence, though, the shock of parting her hair ever so slightly and then seeing something run at me like an angry bull charging through a follicular field was too much to take. That said, I managed to pull it back and, in one of my proudest moments, treated her first. Genuinely, totally thought if it ever happened to me it'd be like a plane crash 'SAVE YOURSELVES' scenario where you put the oxygen mask on before sorting the kids. A mother's love right there. Tell you what, they're persistent little shits. Absolutely refused to die. Two things that would survive an apocalypse: canned pineapples and nits. We tried everything – holistic approaches and all the chemicals. Nothing resulted in the instantly itch-free feeling I was hoping for. A personal highlight was Steve romantically massaging Full Marks solution into my scalp from the toilet seat, as I sat in between his legs, parodying Patrick Swayze and Demi Moore in a greasier version of *Ghost*. Eventually, after what felt like months of regular wet combing with conditioner and my salty tears of despair, we were finally free of the little fuckers. The mental scars and PTSD (Post Traumatic Scratch Disorder), however, live on. I'm constantly on an itchy edge … What if I didn't get them all? What if they come back? I'm half woman, half chimpanzee, constantly rooting around in the kids' heads looking for signs, legs, and eggs. Absolutely horrific, I'm not sure there could be anything worse …

Wait, what now? Parasitic beings that live and breed in your arsehole? Poke their heads out in the dead of night to deliver eggs like a demonic and bloodsucking easter bunny! NO. FUCKING. THANK YOU.

Question: why aren't intestinal worms on the national curriculum? We should all be taught about these silent ass-assins in high school, mainly as a form of birth control, but also so we all have informed choices about our futures. Parents need more information, like when we had daily Covid briefings. I want to know what the 'R … se' number is like in my area – screw a national code red, we need to be on a code brown. Should the kids' nails be clipped back like a cat's claws? Do we need to get to higher ground? We need help! Fortunately, we're yet to have them … well, that I know of. They could be in there right now, couldn't they? Tucking into last night's chicken nuggets. If I screamed at head lice, think it's fairly safe to say I'd literally lose my shit over bum worms. Also, the Sunday date-night nit comb seems hugely preferably to laying on your back and passing your other half a torch. Never mind 'until death us do part', more like 'until our arse cheeks do part'. We always tell kids things to scare them, for their own good. Don't cross a road without looking – you'll get run over. Don't talk to strangers – it's five minutes of your life you'll never get back. Tell you what we don't use enough

… worms. Don't scratch your arse then put your fingers in your mouth – otherwise gigantic arse-tunnelling aliens will eat your chocolate brioche from the inside. Sleep tight, little ones, don't let the bum bugs bite!

Yes, your child's journey into education is a big old adjustment, for everyone. It's a chance for them to be independent, meet new friends (which they absolutely will), and do all the fun arty things you never let them do at home. It can also be a daunting new prospect … being separated from you, having to wipe their owns bums, and, if you're my daughter, the ultimate punishment – a school dinner. It's a pretty exhausting process for them too, although I'm not entirely sure why … you didn't hear Dolly Parton singing about working '9 To 3' – they aren't exactly putting a big shift in, are they? Have school days always been this short? I just about manage to take my coat off and plough through their snacks before I'm off out again to collect them. Tell you what is tiring, the sheer amount of things parents have to remember – the dress-up days, homework, reading books, harvest festival tins, empty cardboard boxes – it's enough to make you want to lie down in a dark room and weep for your long lost twenties. Nothing will ever beat the panic of waking up at 2 a.m. and realising it's a PE day but the kit isn't clean. I'd like to say school gets easier as they get older, but so far it's looking like it gets worse. The homework becomes more frequent and difficult. Also, their inclination to do it wavers, and with them weighing roughly half of your own body mass, it becomes increasingly harder to pick them up and plonk them down at a table to do it. There will be tears, tantrums, refusals to get out of bed, and playdates with kids who, despite telling their parents they were an absolute joy to have, you will never invite round again. Then just like that, in the blink of an eye, it'll all be over … they'll be in high school and you'll be having a breakdown about potential Bunsen burner injuries and teenage pregnancies.

All you'll have to remember those special younger days by is seven years' worth of gurning class photos that look as though someone's holding a gun to their heads, a scrapbook filled with precious memories … and of course, SHART. Lots, and lots, of SHART.

16

The Circle of Strife

As an adult, you think you know things. You may not possess the IQ of a Mensa member, but you clawed your way through the education system, don't do too badly at pub quizzes (while cheating on your phone) and can make a toastie without setting the house on fire. The minute you have kids, however, your base level of intellect is challenged somewhat … Not only is it incredibly apparent you know nothing about youngsters, as a species, but when it comes to imparting your wisdom onto their sponge-like and highly inquisitive little minds, you very quickly realise … you don't know shit about shit. Quite often, this eye-opening comprehension comes when said children start getting older, begin taking more notice of the world around them, and start using their newly acquired language skills to constantly interrogate you about some of life's more challenging aspects …

'What day did God create the dinosaurs?'

'If oranges are called oranges because they're orange, why aren't bananas called yellows?'

'What's 765 million times 6033?'

'When you cry, is it your eyes going for a wee?'

'What's that smell?'

'It's Mummy … on the toilet. GO AWAY!'

Questions, questions, and more questions. Our kids plague us with them morning, noon and night – especially at night because it's an excellent tactic for delaying sleep and for holding a poor unsuspecting parent hostage for an extra hour, while their dinner goes cold. Generally speaking, I can't escape the evening routine without enduring lengthy interrogations about the universe so complex even the great Stephen Hawking would have struggled to answer them. 'A Brief History of Pissing About at Bedtime' would have been more fitting. Yes, there's nothing quite like having kids to remind you of the fact you really should have worked harder at school.

'Mummy, what happens when a star dies?'

'Errr … a Twitter hashtag, and then the *Daily Mail* exposes all of their secrets. Night night!'

In most scenarios, the internet will be your saviour, along with your two best, and wisest, friends – Alexa and Siri. How on earth did parents respond to the onslaught of questions from the Spanish Kidquisition prior to the invention of the world wide web? Well, I can hazard a guess … they didn't, which is probably why we're all now as thick as two short planks. If it's not time and space, it's mathematical calculations, the anatomy of made-up creatures, and my daughter's personal favourite (normally reserved for motorway driving, in pissing-down rain) – colour chemistry. 'What would we get if we mixed flamingo pink with a hint of rich mauve, a dash of fridge-exposed Avocado green, gone-off-mince maroon, and 5 ml of dog-piss yellow?'

'A big mess! Now be quiet before we crash into a very brown and green tree!' In reality, you never know the answer – the only thing Mummy is good at mixing is gin. The good news here is there's zero pressure to ever take her to Disneyland – a trip to the B&Q paint-mixing desk will suffice.

Now, some questions are tough because you had way too much fun at university … and others are tough because you know the answer will completely shatter their precious and highly protected beautiful innocence forever. In the very early years of your child's life, you've mostly been responsible for keeping them alive and teaching them to alternate fingers when arse scratching and nose picking. All too soon, however, those highly curious little minds will start to ponder some of life's more emotionally challenging questions, like the circle of life, and you, my friend, are going to have to deal with it to the very best of your parenting abilities.

'Mummy, what happens when we die?'

Death, oh it's the WORST question! Yet a topic that, from such a young age, they are *totally* fixated on. I get it, it's the great unknown … pretty much every adult still wants to know what happens when their number's up. Do we just slip into an abyss of black nothingness? Or, do we ascend to heaven? Trying to blag our way onto God's VIP list, past St Paul the bouncer – skinhead, white puffer jacket, and tattooed knuckles sporting 'love' on one hand, 'gate' on the other. 'Errr, no my name should definitely be on the list … Sophie with a 'p'. Is Jesus there? He and my dad, John, go way back … oh no, not to Galilee – mainly just to socks-and-sandal wearing. If this is about the dinosaur question, I didn't answer it, OK? Alexa did!' Or, are we dragged down to the fiery bowels of hell, destined to an eternity of torture and PPI calls for being generally shit humans, using way too many plastic straws, and committing arguably the biggest sin of all … saying the word 'amazeballs'?

A lot of your children's questions about the great beyond will no doubt have been spurred on along by fun old Uncle Walt – everyone's favourite parent-murdering, family movie time buzzkill. 'Where's her mummy? Why's his daddy not moving? Why has that man shot the nice deer? Why? Why? WHY?!' FYI, when you see 'PG' next to a Disney film, it means 'Parents Gone'; skip it and move on to something more cheery – *Game of Thrones*, or *The Texas Chainsaw Massacre*, for example. They're a bit dark, aren't they? Opening scene of *Finding Nemo* … casual murder of his mother and not one, but 4,000 of his siblings. Did they all have to die? Could we not have had the same 'persevere in the face of adversity' moral of the story if Nemo just wandered off in Aldi for twenty minutes? Marlin could have found him the middle aisle holding a giant chorizo ring and debating the need for a foil insulation blanket and a new cat bed – would have been far less upsetting. Then there's *Frozen* … orphaned sisters, and plenty of parents now put off ever embarking on a cruise to the Norwegian fjords. Maybe a safari would be better? Apart from all the wildebeest stampedes, that is … *Hakuna Matata*! It means no worries, for the rest of your days! Unless you're five, and now having repetitive nightmares about Daddy being mowed over by a herd of cows.

Jack was only about three or so when he first raised the question of his own mortality after one of his toys broke, asking me with the biggest, saddest eyes 'Mummy, what happens when my batteries run out? Will I not work any more?' I'm not crying, you are! It was awful. Managing to spout off some bollocks about him having special ones that were rechargeable and would never run out, I then locked myself in the bathroom and wept uncontrollably. 'Mummy's OK, she's just having a tricky poo!'

You come to realise death is everywhere, and you can't shield them from it forever. All too soon you'll be faced with a splattered bunny on the road, and no matter how good Duracell are, it ain't going to get up and keep going. And so it begins ... the great 'afterlife' hard sell. Cat-mauled pigeons get repatriated up into bird heaven; there's also stood-on-spider heaven ... bumble bee heaven ... hedgehog heaven ... and fictional cat heaven (big shout out to Judith Kerr for killing off Mog). It really does break your heart watching their little minds process the information that life is finite, that we have a start ... and an end point. Your expiration date, in particular, is of great interest to your now morbidly obsessed children. As soon as they're aware of death as a concept, your card is marked, but not in an overly concerned 'I love you so much, can't live without you' kind of way. No. It's more of a 'need to diarise the event so it doesn't clash with *Peppa Pig*' way.

'Mummy, when exactly *are* you going to die? Tomorrow? Two months, 1,500 days?' You weren't planning on croaking that soon but now you're beginning to wonder if you've given them homicidal ideas. Ohhh, they want all the gory details, along with an exact schedule and timeline of your grisly demise. When, where, how? You're fucked if you've got a wrinkle too ... they're pretty much ready to read you your last rites. My poor friend Amy came to visit from Australia and her face hadn't been given the chance to rehydrate properly from the flight before my two Grim Reapers descended on her. 'What are those lines on your head? Are they because you're old? Are you going to die soon?' The fear of them being around the actual elderly is unreal – you never quite know what they're going to say, much like the Queen probably felt going anywhere with Prince Phillip. Family pets are also fairly disposable, with very little sentiment attached to their short existence on this planet. 'Mummy, when is Millie going to doggy heaven?'

'Oh, sweetheart, don't worry – not for a really long time!'

'Oh ...'

'What's wrong?'

'I wanted a puppy ...'

So very brutal. Our dog was raging at their fickleness – you could see it in her eyes, she was plotting her gassy revenge. 'I've had eight years of your shit, pulling my tail, preoccupying my humans, fucking reindeer ears at Christmas and THIS is the thanks I get?'

It wasn't until they were five and three, respectively, that we were faced with our first non-creature or fictional character death – their beloved Great Grandma, 'GiGi'. They absolutely adored her so we steeled ourselves for completely inconsolable and hysterically sobbing children ... Yeah, that didn't quite pan out. Genuinely, there would have been more of an emotional reaction if we'd run out of crisps. Zero fucks given. On asking if they had any questions, Jack replied, 'Yes ... Can I go and play Lego now?' Evelyn, who was happily mixing every colour of Play-Doh she could find into a ball of murky grey, didn't even look up. 'Are you both OK? It's totally normal to feel sad and have a cry ...' I probed, totally freaked out by their lack of reaction, while simultaneously crafting a homemade crucifix out of pipe cleaners. The power of Christ compels you! Jack, who eyeballed me as though I was a right thicko, said (rather condescendingly), 'But she's in heaven now ...'

'With the pigeons!' Evelyn piped up.

'So we'll just see her when we get there!' He concluded. And that was that. Off he popped to carry on building his Lego satanic altar. No tears, no hours of questioning. Nada. Obviously, this set me off into an absolute downward spiral of parental panic. Smoke was coming out of my computer keyboard with the speed I was googling 'early warning signs of psychopaths'. Also, what if something happened to me, and Steve had to tell them I'd died, would they be like, 'Cool, she's up there doing her things as the bird lady from *Home Alone 2*. What's for tea?' NOTHING, BECAUSE MUMMY'S DEAD

AND DADDY STILL DOESN'T KNOW HOW TO TURN ON THE OVEN!

I've since spoken to quite a few people who've had similar nonchalant responses from kids in the face of bereavement, and it seems it's just the way their brains process things – so very different to how an adult would comprehend such a dramatic life event. To them, death is not permanent – especially with the notion of an all-singing, all-dancing heaven that many parents portray – so why should they be upset? Their minds are still full of such magic and wonder – to them, nothing is impossible, even the thought of someone coming back to life. Though we'd explained Gigi was gone, multiple times, Evelyn would still continue to ask when she'd be visiting from heaven, or if we were going to see her for Christmas and what gift she'd bring us, and how old she'd be on her next birthday. Jack too would occasionally drop random, and very matter-of-fact, death-related statements into conversation; for example, on the phone to Steve's mum he'd say, 'Hi! Your mum is dead!' Or to total strangers, including the lady at the McDonald's Drive-Thru, 'My GiGi died!' Er, we'll have some chicken nuggets with a side order of awks, please. Even though they hadn't initially reacted to the news, you could tell they were both still mulling it over in their little minds, trying to make sense of it all. It wasn't until a few months later, after a mummy-fail of epic proportions, they both gained further, and somewhat unwelcome clarity on the matter. NB this is a lesson on how NOT to explain the process of death to small children. There's a very good reason why this book is not a parenting manual, more of a safe space of collective fuck-ups that'll make you feel a bit better about your own abilities ...

Brace yourselves, it's pretty bad ... So, Evelyn's ballet class is held in a church hall, and to get there we have to walk through the graveyard. We were running ten minutes late (standard) when Jack decided it would be a great time to ask what all the rectangles in the ground were for. Now, in the stress inducing rush of the moment, the question was *potentially* answered a little too flippantly.

'Oh, they're just where you go when you die!' Well ... the absolute horror, because there he stood, as dead in his tracks as the people six feet under. 'YOU SAID WE GO TO HEAVEN WHEN WE DIED!'

Uh oh ...

'Wait ...' he reflected, 'DO YOU CLIMB INSIDE OF THEM TO DIE?'

'Not unless you want to get buried alive!' I VERY, very wrongly jested. It was not the time for jokes.

'YOU. CAN. GET. BURIED. ALIVE?'

It was at that moment I realised it was going to be very difficult to a) claw this back, b) get them to sleep at any point in the next six years, and c) explain to a police officer why two small, and crying, children were being dragged through a graveyard at 6 p.m. on a dark winter's night. In trying to smooth over the situation, there was a misjudged attempt at trying to make things slightly better by explaining you didn't *actually* die in the grave unless you were very unlucky, but somewhere else first like a hospital, your house, or even a car!

'A CAR?! I don't want to die in our car Mummy! Is it going to happen now, on the way home from ballet?' Unlikely. We'd still be stood in that exact same spot fifty-six years later, me badly answering questions and him still absolutely refusing to get in Mummy's Happy-Meal-box and banana-skin-strewn shit tip death-mobile.

'But Mummy, why *do* people need graves if they go to heaven?' A valid point I wasn't quite prepared for, and while stumbling around trying to find a non-traumatising answer we inadvertently ventured down an even more confusing avenue.

'Well … your body stays here, but your soul goes to heaven.' Yep … shoved a stick of dynamite into the question equivalent of Pandora's box – blew it WIDE open.

'What's a soul?'

Now, maybe it *could* have been described as the incorporeal and immortal essence of living beings … a psyche that includes consciousness, reason, memory, perception and feelings. I, obviously, opted for a more simplified version of 'It's just something that lives inside you!'

'LIKE WORMS?'

'Errr no … not worms. It doesn't live in your bum, but your head …'

'WHAAAAAAAAAAT?' He gasped in horror. 'YOUR BODY STAYS ON EARTH BUT YOUR HEAD GOES TO HEAVEN?'

Shit.

'NO!! No. You don't get decapitated … that's just a type of coffee that doesn't keep you awake. It's … it's … more of a *gas* that gets released when you die, which then floats up to heaven …' He looked at me, those big blue eyes wide with bewilderment, and whispered …

'Like a *fart*?'

'Yes …' I replied. 'Your body stays on earth but your farts go to heaven. LET'S GO!'

Finally, it was time for us all to move onto a better place … Nando's. Ballet finished hours ago. Stomachs full of dead chickens ('Mummy what are chickens made out of …'), we headed for home – Evelyn crying her eyes out at the new information we eat fluffy animals, and also because she wanted her farts to stay on earth with Mummy and Daddy. Driving back to our house, Jack had one last parting question …

'Mummy, can we see Gigi's grave?'

'No, sweetheart, she was cremated!' I replied, without engaging ONE single brain cell, and as soon as those words tumbled out of my mouth, the cruel hand of doom was upon me.

'CREMATED? *WHAT DOES THAT MEAN?*'

You go into a big oven, then set on fire until all that is left is fillings and dust. Sweet dreams!

Scraped knees, hugs, endless love, projectile vomiting, bedtime stories and knowing which dial turns the grill on – I'm a grade-A, gold medallist, parenting winner. Explaining life's tricker questions – as we've established, not my forte. So, you can only imagine how this next conversation went down.

'Mummy, where do babies come from?'

'Errr, where do you think babies come from?'

'Don't know … Shall we ask Siri?!'

'NO!!'

Yes – babies. Another common curiosity for kids, especially older ones, and even more so after they're delivered the news they're about to be delivered ~~competition~~ siblings. When quizzed on the topic, most sensible parents either attempt a straightforward divert, or head to a series of well-rehearsed lies. 'The stork', 'Under a cabbage patch', 'The work's Christmas party …' for example. Never one to make life easy for myself, and guilty about adding yet another fib to the expanding list of Father Christmas, the Easter Bunny, and what tampons are ('What's that string, Mummy?'), I was like, 'Kids, settle down and let me tell you all about the birds and the bees!'

Now, first off, let me tell you all something about the birds and the bees – it's not as it sounds, which would be a Kama Sutra logistical nightmare … BIRDS DON'T SHAG BEES! Which would explain why you don't see stripy seagulls dive-bombing people for chips and then shitting honey all over cars. Opting out of pollination and instead into an arable farming analogy, I thought relatively innocent 'seed' planting metaphors might be easier ground. Daddies have seeds – fairly accurate – which they then plant in mummies (glossing over the ploughing) and then a baby grows! My non-inquisitive, gullible son was totally fine with this explanation – there were zero questions on the matter. My highly suspicious, curiously minded daughter, on the other hand, wasn't buying it. She needed to know the literal ins and outs of the sowing process. 'But how *does* the seed get *into* you, Mummy? Does Daddy put it in your mouth and then you swallow it?' Errr, Daddy wishes … Unaware, at the point of explanation, that she'd been growing runner beans at school (so knew some of the basics required for successful sprouting) she was very excited at the prospect of Daddy getting his hands dirty in Mummy's garden. 'He needs to keep your soil nice and wet!' she chirped. Absolutely bloody horrifying. Changing tack, before the word 'moist' came into play, I opted instead for every child's favourite thing … magic! There is one thing, sadly, kids enjoy more than magic and that's asking questions about magic. 'Did Daddy pull out his wand? Did he say the magic word? Did he have an assistant? Did his friends Ron and Hermione turn up and join in? Did he have to go to a special school? Did you get to ride a special train? CAN YOU TALK TO SNAKES?!' Moving swiftly away from Sprogwarts, the marginally more ambiguous explanation of a 'special cuddle' was explored …

'Like the special cuddles we give Grandad?'

'Noooooooooooo! Absolutely not.'

'Like the special cuddles Daddy gives Millie dog?' Oh, dear God, Mummy really hopes not – although he is partial to a bit of doggy …

'It's more a special kiss' I tried to differentiate.

'Were you and Daddy making a baby in the kitchen earlier?' Again, Daddy wishes …

With the kids more confused than ever, and me terrified they might go into school and tell their teachers they saw their parents shagging over Shredded Wheat, it was time to enlist the help of external resources – in the form of educational books. WELL, what a bloody eye-opener they were – for me, that is. Some of the illustrations! Wowsers. Bit graphic. Also made me feel about as sexually adventurous as a rock. One book had stick people bonking on a space hopper. A SPACE HOPPER? How does that work from a logistics standpoint without someone ending up in A&E? I'm all for honesty and transparency, but the kids don't need to know Daddy drilled Mummy over an inflatable. In the end, I chose a non-illustrated version of the truth … men have magical time-and space-travelling tadpoles that teleport into a woman's tummy after she's asked him to take the bin out. Done.

'But Mummy, how do the babies come out?'

'Errr, they come out of tummies, or minnies …'

'IS THAT WHAT THE STRING'S FOR?'

Here's the thing – prenatal classes don't always equip you with the skills required for parenting in the real world. Parenting is sometimes a constant panicked balance of trying to protect your child's innocence, but also ensuring they're savvy enough in life that when they're 25 they aren't highly suspicious of frogs. In an ideal world, I'd keep them little, completely ignorant, and locked in my cellar forever. When you sign up for motherhood, no one tells you how to do all this stuff! It's only when you're in the thick of it, shouting at your kids to stop screaming the word 'sperm' at the top of their lungs in the middle of Tesco, you realise it's mostly about trial and error. In my case, lots of error.

Am I a perfect parent? No. Am I parent who mostly just wings it? Sure! Am I a parent who'll be paying for therapy for my kids' fear of amphibious creatures for the next fifteen years – abso-fucking-lutely! You can only do your best, what you feel is right at the time, and of course … you could always just ask Siri.

Oh, and with the tampon thing … NEVER TELL THEM IT'S A MOUSE.

17

Mother's Day

I am led to believe there is a female equivalent to Father's Day ... where us gals receive copious bunches of flowers, get to relax with our feet up, and finally catch up on some sleep ... I believe it's called death.

When it comes to Mother's Day, expect nothing, then be pleasantly surprised when handed a still-wet-with-PVA homemade card your other half has forced the kids to make five minutes earlier.

It's just like EVERY. OTHER. FUCKING. DAY. Mentally prepare your revenge, and move on.

18

The Mile Cry Club

Do you remember in your youth when holidays were carefree, STI-risking, 18–30s trips to Greek islands? When days would consist of sun worshipping, margarita drinking, and sleeping round the pool for hours at a time then waking up sporting third-degree burns and resembling a Drumstick lollipop? Evenings – oh, they were all about getting dolled up and making bad life choices, weren't they? You'd down fishbowls, throw up fishbowls, dance until dawn then get up at midday ready to do it all over again. Ah, the good old days.

But hey, life is a little different now and travelling to foreign countries with young children is also fun … SAID NO PARENT EVER. Despite this, millions of us overly optimistic parents choose of our own free will to break free from the mumdane and make the treacherous warm-weather pilgrimage abroad for our annual 'helliday'.

Preparation for the summer shit show actually starts a year prior to setting one buniony, flip-flopped foot on burning sand. Yes, the quest for a 'perfect' family vacay is as long as it is gruelling, because when kids are in tow it's just not as easy as picking a Teletext three-star apartment in Kavos. No, there is a very specific list of demands that must be met for maximum enjoyment/bearability. For example, is it child-friendly? Have 25,000 neurotic individuals left a minimum of a four-star TripAdvisor rating for it? Is there a must-have tacky pirate ship in a non-slip, urine-filled swimming pool? And MOST importantly … is there a kids' club that takes children over the age of three? That, my friend, is an ABSOLUTE game changer – the four-leaf clover of hotels. Very rare to find, and you're lucky as fuck if you manage to get in. Also, without fail, every year you still want to be within walking distance of bars and restaurants … but why, though? Where do you think you're going? Raving? God loves a trier – you go ahead and enjoy a bit of 'I can't get no sleep' … but it'll be in your hotel room at 4 a.m., crying toddlers hanging off your neck because the bed/pillow/smell/water/air is different. One thing that becomes apparent about holidays as a parent is that they are no longer about you – they're about the kids and making precious, precious memories … shouting at them repeatedly for cannonballing elderly people in the swimming pool. 'DO THAT AGAIN AND I'M TAKING AWAY YOUR DEVICES!' A wholly empty threat, and they know it, because without the electric babysitters there would be no holiday for parentkind. The only option for you is to *not* follow through on the punishment, retreat to your sun lounger and neck a pina colada while listening to the shrieks of partially drowned and blinded-by-chlorine pensioners.

It takes so long to deliberate between which overpriced, feral-child-filled complex to visit that by the time you come to book, nothing's available – forcing you to choose a holiday that fulfils only 10 per cent of your checklist of requirements, but at the time the thought of being warm and scoffing Jamon Ruffles blocks out any rational judgement.

For family holiday newbies, let me give you an invaluable piece of advice here … NEVER tell your children you are going away until the morning it's actually happening – your sanity and eardrums can thank me later.

'Mummy, how many days until we go on holiday?'

'236, sweetheart … Same number of days as this morning, and at three-minute intervals thereafter.' It's bad enough they have a vague awareness of when Christmas and Easter falls – do not throw holidays into the mix too.

Once you've painfully run down the holiday countdown clock, which will feel closer to 782 days following the constant bombardment of questioning, you can start packing … every item of clothing you've ever bought your children into 20 kg worth of easyJet luggage. How many T-shirts might your slobbery toddler get through? Who the hell knows? Not even the woman, the myth, the legend Carol Vorderman could make that calculation. 'I'll take three from the top and forty-seven from the bottom shelf please, Carol … then just throw in the rest in case of projectile bodily fluids.' And nappies? How many nappies? Is eighteen a day for two weeks going to be enough? It's a well-known fact that the good people of Greece, Spain, Portugal, Turkey, etc. do not have nappies, so what will you do if you run out? For the love of God, WHAT WILL YOU DO?! Once you've shoehorned in lilos, inflatable mythical creatures, and enough spades to dig out a second Channel Tunnel, there's no room for any of your clothes, meaning you'll have to squeeze everything you own into the 10 kg of free cabin baggage reserved for plane snacks. It then becomes a horrific choice between strappy wedges, or the 500 Bear YoYos you know will prevent an international incident at 33,000 feet. You rationalise living in flip-flops for two weeks because, realistically, the only night scene you'll be part of is the mini disco – twerking against a Danish holiday rep in a tiger costume. Seriously, the list of crap you need to take is endless: Calpol, thermometers, baby sleeping bags, car seats, swim nappies, every factor of sun lotion, and an out-of-date tub of Sudocrem in case of an itchy arse. Do you ever have anxiety dreams about trying to fill a suitcase for a flight that's just about to leave, but you haven't finished packing? Welcome to parenting.

Ready for another endurance test? Combine overly excited children with heaving crowds, a very specific deadline, endless queues, and extremely non-patient shouty people checking you for bombs. Hello airport! You'll never experience blood pressure like it. On one of our most recent trips abroad, my heart rate was so elevated that Siri chirped up, 'Sophie, do you require medical assistance?' Yes, yes I do … and someone to kick the buggy through the X-ray machine. You can never collapse them when you need to, can you? Stroller stage fright is real, and always heightened by a queue of 1000 highly irate travellers behind you, along with a stern-looking security person who's about to lose their shit at the next person who's accidentally left liquids in their hand luggage. 'It's only been this way since 2006, dickheads!'

With the pram as broken as your holiday spirits, it's on to the least fun game ever invented – 'taste the cold baby food to prove it's not an explosive'. Be prepared to look super shifty during this 'am-bush-tucker trial' because you are not OK shovelling down cold pureed sweet potato/whatever wasn't off in the vegetable drawer. Your child can eat it, but there's no way you're putting that mush in your mouth. While you're being strip-searched because of a Minions 'fart blasting' gun someone snuck into your hand luggage, unaccompanied children will have legged it through the metal detectors at speed, and will be attempting to board a flight that is not yours. The distance your mini-Kevin

McCallisters will have managed to cover will be highly dependent on whether or not you've aided and abetted their escape with a vehicle. Ahhh, Trunkies – cute, aren't they? On a shelf in your garage, collecting dust. If you've decided to take one to an airport, more fool you. What they didn't show on *Dragons' Den* was out-of-control children ramming into strangers' Achilles tendons at 50 mph, while parents screech apologies from 100 metres behind. Oh help, oh no … it's a Gruffalo … on bastard wheels.

After telling your kids the pilot won't let them on unless they've had a wee, and risking life and limb lugging a pram, two Trunkies, and kids down six flights of stairs, you can finally board the plane … but not before you and your partner have another argument at the bottom of the stairs about how to collapse the buggy. With the pram broken in several more places and resembling a giant squashed grasshopper that's bleeding a river of apple juice onto the tarmac, you can find your seats … scattered randomly all over the plane. Of course they are. For some unbeknown reason, the budget airline has decided to seat your small child at the back of the plane next to a teenage couple who are about to get a harsh life lesson on the importance of contraception. After a game of musical plane chairs, and your heroic partner 'taking one for the team' sitting at the back of the plane on his own (and already asleep), the seatbelt sign is on and it's time for take-off. Hurrah! Sit back, relax and ease yourself into the holiday spirit … GIN. It's 8.45 a.m. and you're about to embark on a painful four-hour flight to Greece with Cry'an Air. But it's fine … it's FINE. It was your life choice to have children, and you wouldn't have it any other way, repeatedly, explaining to kids who've been up for five hours the importance of tray tables needing to stay in the upright position for take-off. 'Why? So if the plane skids off the runway, sweetheart, we don't all smash our skulls in on them before slowly burning to death. Rice cake?'

Having been delayed at the end of the runway for forty-five minutes and unable to break free for the toilet or reserve snacks, you're up! Everyone is finally happy ... for five minutes, until the novelty of being on a plane wears off and the kids are screaming as though they've been thrown in the Saturday night drunk tank. Arms are being windmilled, a head's bounced off a tray table – 'SEE! They're dangerous!' – and there's been great offence taken at the fact they're not allowed to fly the plane (how very unreasonable). The good news is you've run out of biscuits, the iPad is dead and there's still three hours to go. Somewhere above France you threaten that if they don't pipe down, the pilot's going to turn the plane around and take them home. It doesn't work, so you end up spending a fortune on the world's smallest tub of Pringles to placate them. In my personal experience, kids seem to enjoy the idea of transportation better than the reality. 'Look, Mummy, a plane!' Put them on one and it's a completely different kettle of fish. As they're clambering for the emergency exit, mid-flight, you realise how interchangeable your role of a mother is with that of a nightclub bouncer. I'm semi with them, though, because I hate flying – stepping on that aircraft is essentially akin to a death sentence for me, and repeatedly humming the *Peppa Pig* theme tune while playing I-spy with a child who tells you what they can see before you've even guessed feels like a terrible way to go.

As the plane makes its final descent towards your destination, there's the inevitable twenty minutes of 'my ears hurt' sobbing, which could have been easily avoided if all the lollipops hadn't been annihilated before leaving British airspace. While you're badly trying to explain/demonstrate other ways of clearing your ears, a child wets themselves and you realise you've forgotten to pack spare clothes. Knickers drying on the seat in front, and your child dressed in the only nice top you've brought for yourself – stuffed in your hand luggage – there's just enough time for a lengthy debate as to why window blinds need to be open for landing. 'THEY JUST DO!' Having been desperate to get off the plane for the past four hours and forty-five minutes, suddenly no one wants to leave the cylindrical horror chamber of farts and crumbs, resulting in you having to rugby tackle them off. In doing so, you try not to catch the eye of every other passenger who, thanks to you, has also had the flight from hell. Oh well, at least you can speedily exit the airport and never see them again. Oh wait ... of course your bags were last off the plane, the buggy went AWOL, and one of the kids ricocheted their forehead off the luggage carrousel and had to be tended to by medics.

Walking onto your coach, an hour and a half later, you're greeted by all the happy faces from your flight. Brilliant. They hate you, and to be fair ... it's perfectly understandable. Things couldn't get any worse, could they? Of course they could. Your accommodation is an hour's transfer from the airport, something which at the point of booking didn't really seem *so* much of a big deal but as you feel the warmth of your child's urine flowing through your clothes, down onto the seat and floor below, you realise it is. It *really* is. Having spent the best part of fifty minutes playing reservation roulette (pulling up to shitty-looking hotels and praying they're not yours), you eventually arrive – hot, crumpled, knackered, and smelling of wee. Fortunately, you picked a very classy hotel that has kindly given you a lovely cold flannel to cool down with, which, unfortunately for you, your smallest family members are using to wipe their genitals.

The first few days of the holiday are all about easing yourself in gently ... to all the potential things that could kill your child. Slippy tiles, sharp edges, deep swimming pools, easy to open balcony doors, uncut buffet grapes, and child-hooligans who keep chokeholding your babies under the water as part of a sadistic drowning game. Officially labelled '*that* family' by fellow guests, thanks to your children's foghorn gobs, if you haven't bellowed 'STOP SCREAMING!' at the top of your lungs, apologised to multiple people on their behalf, or had to count to three really slowly at the side of the pool only for your children to ignore you anyway, are you even actually on holiday?

Something you probably never really appreciated before having kids, especially on holiday, was the ability to leave a room quickly. You've had breakfast, you've got your bikini on and you just decide to leave … easy as that. Grab your book, sunnies, phone, bag, sun cream – and leave. Done. Cut to ten years and two sprogs later and exiting your hotel room/villa/prison cell is quite possibly one of the most challenging experiences of your adult life. Not one single fucker has any sense of urgency surrounding the fact it's 30°C outside and Mummy has lumps of flesh she wants to hear sizzle like a fajita on a hotplate. Nope, they're all dicking about colouring, asking to play on your phone, engrossed by Greek TV, or having an hour-long bowel movement. You've been up for six hours and still haven't managed to make it to within four feet of a sun lounger, or a pina colada for that matter. *Fuming.* Also, a solid hour of this process has been dedicated to the smothering of factor 50 sun cream on incredibly unwilling participants. They want to go swimming, swing off the pirate ship, run round the pool and crack their skulls open – but sun 'scream'? Oh, that's never going to happen. Resembles mayonnaise, smells of shampoo. No way. Despite VERY in-depth discussions as to why it's required – 'Because you'll go on fire, sweetheart' – there is complete refusal to cooperate. Going out on a limb here – I've never tried, but it's probably easier to catch a chicken and baste it while still alive than it is to evenly apply lotion to anyone under the age of 18.

At 12 p.m. (perfect timing for spontaneous combustion) your half-basted poultry are out of the door, and you can finally chill out on that lounger … LOLS! Gone are the days of being able to lie still and soak up those delicious and highly dangerous rays. No, life now consists (at intervals of approximately every forty-six seconds) of being asked to blow up armbands, get drinks, mop drinks off floors, find snacks, pick snacks off floors, get in the pool, go see the Danish man in tiger costume, and use all your lung capacity to inflate a gigantic floating unicorn. My absolute favourite request, however, has to be 'Mummy, I need a wee!', which normally occurs within four seconds of them being fully submerged in a swimming pool, despite them wholeheartedly promising they didn't need one before entering. After a thirty-minute grapple with a wet swimming costume and mutant-squid-gripping armbands, you chuck them back into the water with hopes firmly set on at least ten minutes of sun worshiping. HA! Your arse merely grazes the lounger before a little foghorn chirps up. 'Mummy, I need a poo!' At least be thankful they've asked because, I promise this, there's NO bigger fear for a parent on helliday than the shame you'll experience of being the family whose kid shat in the pool. Sirens go off, the pool is evacuated like someone liberated a bag of piranhas in there instead of the previous night's buffet food, and solemn-faced lifeguards take it in turns to draw straws to see who gets the grim job of investigating the UPO (Unidentified Pooey Object). Sieve in hand, a traumatised teenager confirms what a very guilty-faced set of parents sitting around the pool already know to be true. CODE BROWN! Out comes the red tape, the pool is sectioned off to protect the crime scene, and disgruntled parents swear under their breath because it means having to take their kids to the next biggest water source … the bastard beach.

Correct me if I'm wrong here, but one of the main holiday criteria you may have attempted to adhere to (aside from kids' club) is your accommodation's proximity to the seaside, aka Satan's sandpit. I do this too … but let's just all take a minute to ask ourselves WHY?! No one actually enjoys it, including small children partially coated in lard. All part and parcel of making those precious memories, though, isn't it? So that in forty years, you can fondly look back at holiday pics from Greece and wonder why you took two giant Scotch eggs to the beach. To save you from yourselves, if it's not too late, let me walk you through how the trip will unfold ...

1. Massively talk up the magical place of sandcastles, shells, and butts – both the cigarette kind, and the elderly perma-tanned man in a thong kind.
2. Drag children, who are desperate to stay at the hotel, on a forty-minute walk in the scorching midday heat.
3. Realise buggies and sand go together like shit in a pool.
4. Remove hot and crying child, who has decided to get in on the bowel movement theme of the day, from their pram and make them walk across 50°C sand.
5. Totally relate with that time Jesus negotiated the Judaean desert for forty days and forty nights. It's been four minutes.
6. Thirty euros for two sun loungers?! Absolutely not. You are British and will lay your towels on the burning hot sand instead.
7. A child disagrees, making their feelings clear while you're attempting the nappy change, flinging its contents across the sand forcing you to leg it over burning coals after a substantially sized pootato croquette.
8. There's so much screaming that you panic there's been a shark attack. The noise is coming from your own crumb-coated children.

9. Snacks are whipped out … then dropped in the sand.
10. The sobbing continues. Everyone is having the most wonderful, special, and memorable time.
11. You introduce screamy children to the sea. It's wet, cold, and the stones hurt their feet. They run from it, and fall face-down into the sand.
12. There's ZERO opportunity to take an Instagram picture captioned #blessed.
13. You need to apply more sun cream to your child–sandpaper hybrid. It's similar to preparing a skirting board for glossing.
14. They fall face-first into the sand.
15. Twenty minutes in, you decide to call it day. Head back to the hotel – repeating steps 5, 4 and 3.
16. Buy kids an ice cream, to plug their wailing pie holes. They drop them in the sand.
17. Arrive at pool-side sweaty, thighs burning from sand chafe, only to find another family has pinched the loungers you bagged at 7 a.m. Irrationally fume about this while lying on the grass getting bitten by ants.
18. Give children iPads, and order yourselves cocktails in varying strengths.
19. Everyone continues to find sand in various orifices for several weeks.
20. Accept that life's a beach.

The only idea worse than a beach trip is a boat trip. Whatever you do … DO NOT DO THIS TO YOURSELF. You'll pay €70 each to spend three hours at sea, everyone yacking into paper bags/all over their feet, kids crying because they want to go home (to England), and the closest you'll get to spotting a dolphin is in the 'luxury lunch' tuna sandwich. Stay by the pool listening to a chorus of 'can I watch something on your phone', and do not move. DO NOT MOVE!

If you think days are difficult, evenings are also challenging. No time to get all done up and fancy-looking because it would mean sacrificing cocktails around the pool at the only time of day that doesn't burn your child's skin to an absolute crisp. Despite booking a family room, there's no bastard bath, so it takes two hours to tackle ice cream-covered, sticky and sandy kids into a shower. They might have spent the whole day splashing each other in the pool, but clean water from a height is UNACCEPTABLE to them. Before your neighbours have the chance to dial down to reception and complain about the noise, you're out of the door – wet hair, patchy sunburn, and twenty-five colouring books, ready to paint the all-you-can-eat buffet red … with pasta sauce. To clarify, before having kids I was NOT an 'all-inclusive' person. I enjoyed evening strolls around towns, taking in the sights and culture, and leisurely deciding which local restaurant or taverna to frequent. Now, with hungry children who'll only eat beige foods hanging off each shoulder, culture can do one. If your kids are very young and you don't fancy spending €20 on food that'll be thrown on the floor, all-inclusive is absolutely the way forward. My kids, generally speaking, are good eaters … until they step foot on foreign soil, then anything containing any nutritional value is considered to contain arsenic.

'It's just a carrot, sweetheart'

'It's weird!'

'It's not weird, it's a carrot. The same type of carrot you eat at home!'

'IT'S WEIRD!!'

Despite most of the fruit and veg they consume back in Blighty having been grown in the country in which they're temporarily residing, the only non-poisonous edibles believed to be safe are bread, chips, pasta (minus the sauce), rice, pizza (with sauce), crisps, crumb-coated 'fingers', and pancakes – a food group widely known as 'bum blockers'. If your kids also fall into this camp, take some comfort in knowing at least there's no danger of them laying an underwater cable in the pool anytime soon. Little Jemima's parents aren't going to be as smug about her spinach consumption tomorrow morning … Having had a relaxing dinner of constantly standing up to replenish the kids' carbs, only enjoying your own food as everyone else is tucking into their desserts, it's mother-freaking MINI DISCO TIME – aka the closest you'll get to Ibiza. Get ready to bust out your best shapes to banging floor-fillers like 'Superman', 'Macarena', and the 'Veo Veo' song (if you don't know it, I hate you). In the evenings, parents can generally be divided into two camps … the ones who try and keep their kids to a normal bedtime routine and so return to the solitary confinement of their rooms, and those who keep them up until stupid o'clock, drip-feeding them Sprite and iPads. One year we attempted to be the first kind of parents … but having spent a night in our open-plan junior suite, locked in the bathroom drinking cans of San Miguel over the bidet so as not to wake the kids, we decided there was more to life than cracking open a tinny over something people use to wash their cracks. We became the people whose feral children ran around until 11 p.m., shitfaced on sugar and twatting each other because of a disagreement over YouTube. You won't be on your own with this, and after a couple of days, you'll have scouted out some like-minded holiday friends/drinking buddies around the swimming pool. Fellow Brits are generally easy to locate – they'll be the only people attempting to sunbathe on a rainy day. 'You can still catch it through the clouds!' You'll know they're your sort of people if they too are dead behind the eyes, and are letting their kids eat a Magnum at 9.30 a.m. Men will normally befriend each other first, while hiding from their partners and children at the bar all day. The mums will find common ground in burning the shit out of their backs in the toddler pool. You'll be best buds for two weeks … talking about the weather back home, the weather where you are, and how much fun you'll all have when you meet up back in the UK. You will never see those people again.

Just in case it was not evident from the above reading material, going on holiday with young kids is NOT a holiday. I repeat, NOT a holiday. When you get back, three stone heavier, ten years older and the proud guardians of severely constipated children, people will ask 'Did you have a lovely relaxing time?' A RELAXING TIME?! You haven't just returned from a luxury spa break. The only thing that relaxed was your sphincter after the laxative effect of brushing your teeth with foreign tap water/too many Pina Coladas. Potentially I'm being a little bit harsh … no one likes a negative Nancy, after all. It's not all bad, there are some lovely bits too – it's just bloody hard work (although, not as hard as camping). Being on high alert for head injuries, drowning, sand ingestion and sun radiation takes its toll, but I do think we probably underestimate how much enjoyment our kids get from spending quality time away with us. For them, it's just days and days of endless fun – an opportunity to interact with us one-on-one, when we're not constantly telling them 'In a minute!' For a change, we actually have a minute. In fact, we have endless minutes because holidays are a rare chance to put normal life on hold and actually appreciate how much better they've got at swimming, or how much faster they can run, or how much more intricate their little drawings of your fat rolls and wrinkles are. Our computers are packed up, our out-of-offices are on, and all our energy is directed at them. Whether it's being thrown around in the pool, building a sand castle, staying up late, or allowing them to have two ice creams in one day – they're absolutely living their best lives, and really, at the end of the day, isn't that all that matters? Happy sun-kissed faces, endless giggles, and memories that will last a lifetime … good job you'll have those as you'll be hard pushed to get an actual photograph. It's a well-known fact that on holiday all children lose the ability to stay still, look at a camera with both eyes simultaneously, or smile in a way that wouldn't qualify them for the World Gurning Championships.

When you eventually arrive home, if you haven't uttered the words 'I need a holiday to get over my holiday' then, quite frankly, you haven't done it properly.

19

Jack's Mum

One of the most unexpected outcomes of the journey from being 20 and on the dance floor, to 30 with no pelvic floor, is the realisation that having finally and painfully crawled towards adulthood, you've completely lost yourself along the way. Life is totally unrecognisable to how it was before, and there's no going back for you. Stuck in a one-way IKEA system, humming theme tunes to kids' TV programmes, and habitually pointing out ducks, cats and trains even when unaccompanied by your child, you wonder WHAT HAS HAPPENED TO YOUR LIFE?

Here's the thing, though – sometimes you have to go a little off piste before you are rescued …

The loss of my identity was something I really grappled with. Who was I? What was I good at? Aside from pulling off last-minute World Book Day costumes, and hiding vegetables into the blended food of nutritionally suspicious children? And, was being a full-time mum enough for me? Post-kids, everything changed – my mind, body, social life, finances, and even my marriage. In the early days, so immersed by the unyielding clutches of motherhood, there were times I allowed it to completely devour me whole – to the point where it felt as though no fragment of my former self remained. Looking in the mirror, there was little recognition of the person staring back – dark circles under the eyes, thinning hairline, deflated boobs, and non-rectifiable scarred bits. Never feeling as though I had any time to myself from 7 a.m. until 7 p.m., in the evenings I clung to the quietness of the house and my mind, staying up until stupid o'clock in the morning in a bid to claw back some form of control over my day. A combination of exhaustion, constantly being pawed by demanding little hands, and a sense of uncomfortableness in my new body was wreaking havoc – especially on my libido which was more interested in the prospect of a cliff dive than a muff dive. I wished, more than anything, there was a switch that could be flicked in order to feel 'normal' again.

I'd never really had issues with self-esteem prior to this stage of my life, but that's probably because I wasn't permanently followed about by unintentionally observational children with a *Catchphrase* 'say what you see' view of the world. 'Mummy, my front bottom is so much cuter than yours!' Harsh but fair. Cute it is not – definitely less wide-eyed woodland creature, and more ferocious matted bear. One that does not enjoy being poked. 'Mummy, what are all those lines on your head?' 'Laughter lines …' 'What are all those rolls on your tummy?' 'Lard lines …' Birthdays are also fun when your children innocently like to remind you how much closer you are to death 'Mummy, you are SO old now! Are you going to die soon?' Jack gets very confused as to why grown-ups don't have birthday parties like kids do, asking one year 'is it because you don't have any friends?' An actual social recluse, immediately my defensive side came out.

'I have lots of friends ... Ralphie's mummy, Alex's mummy, Elizabeth's mummy ...'

'Why are all of your friends my friends' mummies?'

'BECAUSE YOU ARE MY ENTIRE LIFE!'

When Jack started school, there were mums in the playground who I'd speak to at every drop-off and pick-up, yet I didn't have a clue what their names were for about two years, nor did they know mine – they were simply 'Abbie's mum' or 'Bobby's mum' and I was just 'Jack's mum'. We were nameless entities, floating through life and the playground with the sole purpose of shipping our kids to birthday parties and after school activities, keeping them alive via the medium of snacks. When being called over by a teacher for the dreaded and hushed 'chat' at the door, 'Jack's mum! Could I have a word please?' I'd have the urge to scream 'I'm Sophie! My favourite drink used to be an Apple VK with three vodka shots, I've been tubing in Laos, have tried weed, and have felt very uncomfortable at a sex show in Amsterdam!' Retrospectively, it probably wouldn't have gone down well – unlike the girl in the red-light district. Some of my closest school mum friends are still logged in my phone as 'Sam – Betsy', or 'Rhian – Finn', upgraded to their actual names, but still unable to shake the identities of their limpet-like children too. Why do we do it? Much like Pinocchio, deep down all we want to be is real fucking people. Our children, although a very large part of our psyche, do not define us. We are separate living entities, with very different dreams and ambitions – they aspire to be footballers or artists, and what we mostly want is twelve hours' sleep and for them to love us forever.

After Evelyn's arrival, I decided to quit work altogether. Financially, it made no sense to have them both in childcare while commuting hours to a job I despised, and that left me with an end-of-month profit of £100. Although pleased to finally see the back of my PR career and spend more time with the kids, there was a part of me that struggled with the notion of being a full-time stay-at-home mum. With Steve's job being considerably more interesting than arse wiping, whenever we'd meet new people they'd all want to know the ins and outs of his line of work, but funnily enough … not mine. When it came to me explaining my chosen career, I'd quietly profess that I was 'just a mum'. Let's all take a minute to appreciate that complete bitch-slap and disservice I just did to myself … *just* a mum. Hmmm. OK. Is it not the hardest fucking job in the world? Granted, people work down mines, fly into space, create life-saving nano-bots, operate on babies, and teach preschoolers – but they get paid for that, people! If motherhood, which is responsible for the continuation of the whole world, was advertised in the local paper, going on the description – how many people would apply?

Job Title: Parent/snack bitch

Reports To: The Parent will report directly to a team of highly unreasonable, incredibly demanding, and selectively hard of hearing descendants of Gollum.

Job Overview: The parent is responsible for the feeding, watering, bathing, arse wiping, clothing, educating, entertaining, healing, life coaching, disciplining, defending, and general keeping alive of all members in their team.

Requirements:

Applicants must

1. be available to work 24/7, for 938.571 weeks (minimum)

2. possess a high tolerance of bodily fluids
3. put others' wants and needs before their own at all times
4. be willing to share their food with the wider team
5. be able to heal an injury with a hug and kiss
6. be happy to complete back-to-back day and night shifts
7. have an immunity to colds, viruses and hangovers OR must be willing to still carry out official duties while hanging out of their arses
8. be a go-getter … of shoes, snacks, tissues, plastic tat, etc.
9. be able to express fake enthusiasm on demand
10. be willing to sacrifice social life, identity, nice holidays, and car cleanliness.

Qualifications: Zero

Salary: Fuck all

Benefits:
Holiday pay – None
Day off on birthday – None
Bonus scheme – As many half-eaten fish fingers as you can eat
Rewards – Unconditional love, endless SHART, and bogies wiped on your clothing

WE ALL WENT THROUGH SOME SERIOUS SHIT TO GET OUR IMPERFECTLY PERFECT HUMAN BEINGS. MANY OF US AQUIRING PHYSICAL AND MENTAL SCARS, OTHERS LOSING THEIR HAIR, SEX DRIVE AND ABILITY TO HOLD DOWN MORE THAN THREE UNITS OF

ALCOHOL. WE ARE COMITTED TO STAYING AWAKE FOR THE REST OF THEIR LIVES WORRYING ABOUT THEM – HAPPY TO SACRIFICE OURSELVES COMPLETELY FOR THEIR HEALTH, HAPPINESS AND HARRY POTTER MERCHANDISE OBSESSION. WE ARE FUCKING INCREDIBLE! JUST A MUM? HOW'S ABOUT 'JUST A MOTHERFUCKING HERO'?!

Life is challenging, but as a straight, white, non-disabled mother, I'm conscious of the fact that life is easier for me than for so many others out there. On top of the already challenging role of motherhood, I'm not constantly fighting for my child's or my voice to be heard, or face to be seen. I'm statistically less likely to die in childbirth than some women, and will not have to worry about my children being subjected to cruel racial slurs or unjust discrimination. One of the biggest hopes I have for my kids is that they'll grow up in a far more tolerant, kinder and equal society – one that not only fully embraces different identities, cultures and religions but wholeheartedly celebrates them too. A huge part of that responsibility falls into my hands, because parenting is so much more than just 'looking after' your kids. We're their influencers, moral fibre, educators, mind-openers and example setters. Yes, it might be one of the hardest, least financially viable positions on the open market, but it is, admittedly, one of the best.

As a twenty-something woman harbouring the maternal instincts of an egg-abandoning snake, there was a genuine worry as to what would happen when my baby arrived. Would I love it, or even like it? Might I consume it if a little too peckish and Steve wasn't fast enough with the snacks, like a postpartum hamster? GOOGLE IT! Horrific.

Fortunately for all concerned, there were instincts, and love! Who knew?! Turns out my kids are two of the best decisions I've ever made in my life – hands down better than the time I tried Sun In, or a DIY bikini wax. It's a crazy, sometimes incredibly overbearing, love that brings out a fairly violent side of me I didn't know existed prior to their arrival. I was once told having children would turn me into a lioness – fearless, confident, powerful, and willing to take on the world in order to protect my young. A few years and two children down the line, I sometimes feel more like a dominated meerkat than queen of the jungle … but if anyone dared lay a finger on them, a raging momgoose would shred them to pieces, feasting on their evil hearts while majestically bathing in mauled and bloodied remains.

It's also brought out a much softer side of me … I cry a lot, mostly when they're asleep, about how much I goddamn love them, or over the fear of anything bad ever happening to them. Tears also uncontrollably pool into my bra, because as well as wanting them to flourish and grow, I'd also like time to stand still and for them to stay tiny, adorable mummy-worshippers forever. Jack has started asking when he can stop calling me Mummy. 'Errr, make like Prince Charles, and never.' Sometimes it's the realisation of how miraculous they truly are that sets me off as well … imagine, if that exact sperm didn't meet that one egg, they wouldn't be the people you couldn't live without. Steve has often found me hysterical at the thought that our children might not have been. 'YOU COULD HAVE WANKED THEM INTO SOCK, BABE!' A parent's love is absolutely the definition of 'unconditional', totally different than that of a partner's – which is affection that comes with a certain amount of pre-agreed caveats. Sometimes I'm not overly convinced my feelings of affection towards my children are entirely reciprocated … I'd like to think so, but then there's also a part of me that worries if they found me dead at the bottom of the stairs they might step over my bloated corpse and head straight to the snack cupboard …

There's a lot to thank my children for. The first is the laughter and happiness they bring to my life; the second is the fact that, finally, at the ages of five and eight they now sleep past 8 a.m. on a weekend; and the third is for the completely different perspective on life they have given me. Never truly comfortable or happy in my job, it was having the headspace away from office life that made me realise how much I categorically never wanted to go back, and that – unknowingly – the time I was spending at home with the kids was actually sparking a whole new career path for me. Having always been of the opinion that if you didn't laugh about certain things in life, then you'd cry (uncontrollably), as a new and completely out of my depth parent there was a constant wealth of material that if it wasn't happening to me would be hilarious. Being used to a certain level of creativity in PR, when the kids were sleeping (pretty much never) or zoned out in front on CBeebies (pretty much always), I started documenting our daily struggles and successes on a blog that I entitled 'Tired N Tested'. It was mainly just an outlet to begin with – something to flex my brain and distract me from the fact there really wasn't much going on outside of my four walls and my local Tesco Express. During the process, it became apparent how much I enjoyed spending time alone (funny that) on the computer, cathartically hammering out words and bringing them to life with what I hoped was a degree of honesty. Truth be told, I'd always fancied being an author – but post-kids, I felt there would never be the time or confidence to pursue that dream. After posting my entries to Facebook, things really began to pick up, with people other than my parents and their 60-year-old neighbours choosing to follow me. At the time, one of my good friends was visiting and convinced me that in order to move things forwards, vlogging was where it was at. Absolutely not, I insisted!

What was I, a 30-year-old mum of two, going to talk about in a video? 'Hey you guys, welcome to my channel! Today I'm going to show you my top ten incontinence-pad looks!' Worried about sounding like an absolute bloody idiot just waffling incoherently to the camera, I decided on much more of a 'wallflower' approach to the situation … an all-singing, all-dancing parenting parody of Ed Sheeran's 'Shape of You', not so creatively named 'Smell of Poo'. Lyrical genius, me! Naturally, it was the obvious choice for a camera-shy and somewhat vocally challenged woman with no prior experience of video editing or singing in tune. Turns out that one decision changed EVERYTHING. Worried it was potentially the biggest fold-yourself-in-half cringefest ever to grace the internet, I very nearly put it straight in the computer's rubbish bin. What was I thinking? But … it was already done, ready to go, and in all reality likely to be seen by 10 per cent of the 400 people who followed me – what was the real harm? Maybe, I might even get 500 followers and an alcohol brand might send me a bottle of gin. It was worth a shot, literally.

Posting it at 2.30 p.m. on Facebook, off I went to collect Jack from preschool, not giving it a second thought until about three hours later, checking to see if it was getting panned by my dad. It was on 100,000 views. Was that good? With Steve away, I cracked on with the bath and bedtime routine, completely unaware of the madness unfolding on the wondrously strange but incredibly confusing internet. By the time the kids were asleep it had already reached the one million views mark, and my phone was POPPING off. Sitting in the kitchen, completely in the dark, and not sure what do next, I opted to panic-eat crumpets and watch in a blind panic as the figures continued to climb and climb and climb. It turns out I'd gone viral, and on that occasion wouldn't be requiring two Imodium and a litre of Lucozade. By the time the video had run its course, the views stood at 25 million. WHAT?! Sheer ludicrousness. I'd been on the local news, radio, and had even been down to the *Good Morning Britain* studio for a DISASTROUS live TV interview with two small and completely unimpressed children (you can still google 'mother's live TV interview gets sabotaged by 4-year-old boy'. FFS). The number of people following me (hopefully on the internet and not from behind bushes) exploded and suddenly, from nowhere, there was an audience eagerly anticipating more. With a platform to share my comedy, combined with all the ups and downs of parenting, there was no going back. It was up to me to take the opportunity and absolutely run with it (not too fast, or I'd piss myself).

Over the next three years I completely threw myself into the brilliant, yet occasionally dark and incredibly frustrating, world of online content creation – turning something that initially started as a bit of a punt into a full-time career. Surprisingly for all involved, I was actually quite good at it. Who knew?! Also, working from home and to my own schedule finally allowed me to a have job that fitted around the kids – no judgemental eyes when finishing early to collect them, no needing to worry about taking time off if one of them was sick. It was a flexible job I'd created by myself, for myself, out of motherhood – and what a feeling that was. From those early days starting out to now, more has changed. I've evolved, found my footing, taken risks and ultimately discovered a part of me I didn't know existed before having kids. The online world has crossed into the real world too – here I am having finally written that book I'd always dreamed of, but never thought possible. More astoundingly, if someone had said to me five years ago that I'd have got on a stage and made people laugh, I'd have presumed it would have been in a pretty disastrous attempt at making it as an exotic dancer … Never in my wildest dreams would I have imagined it would be stand-up comedy. When I was seven or eight, my Uncle Dave once told me I'd make a great comedian – even at that totally fearless point in my childhood my train of thought was, 'Abso-fucking-lutely not, Dave'. Fate and destiny, however, work in mysterious ways and I often wonder whether I'd be doing all these things now if I hadn't taken that gamble of putting my first video online – or if the kids hadn't come along.

Motherhood, although incredibly overwhelming and with the ability to cut through self-esteem and confidence like a hot knife through butter, has provided me with the ability to believe in and push myself harder than I ever thought imaginable. You might feel as though your life has completely changed after having kids, or you may be at the point of jumping off the precipice but worried that if you take the plunge into parenting your life will be over. I'm here to reassure you it's not. Although it may feel that way for a very short time, change is good and with it comes opportunity, new beginnings, and fresh perspective. Putting yourself out there and taking a risk is scary, and there are still times now when I'm like, 'Oh my God, what am I doing?!' both professionally and as a mother, but then I always like to refer back to a time when my legs were in stirrups and I was shitting into the hands of a student midwife, and think that nothing can be worse than that! Sometimes you've just got to take the plunge and ask yourself 'what's the worst that can happen?' If it doesn't result in public defecation, then maybe give it a whirl. We're always encouraging our kids to believe in themselves, telling them that they can do anything they set their minds to (apart from getting the Play-Doh out), but at what age do we stop telling that to ourselves? Bloody believe in yourself, because you are spectacular! People might not laugh at what I do, or they may say horrible things about me online, but it really doesn't matter in the grand scheme of things because it's not what's keeping me awake at night – that's firmly in the hands of my children crawling into my bed at 3 a.m. and asking if they can watch something on my phone.

With the pure joy and sunshine also comes the feeling of knowing no matter how hard we work, however many hours we put in, we'll never ever feel as though we've done enough. Yes, mum guilt – as much a part of the job as raising them and teaching them to wipe front to back. If my crimes were ever read out in court, I imagine proceedings would go down a little like this … 'On the charges of pretending all soft-play centres are closed, stealing money from piggy banks for pay-and-display car parks, telling them all chocolate is spicy, never volunteering at school, being late for everything, and screaming like an animal being mauled by a meerkat from 8 a.m. to 10 p.m., how do you plead?' 'Errr … guilty' I feel this so deeply, about EVERYTHING. For example, the kids and I don't really have that many common interests yet … which makes me feel bad, but on the other hand … not quite bad enough to willingly spend six hours playing Lego. 'Darling, Mummy's already built the building blocks of life – you crack on while I Instagram-stalk an ex-boyfriend from fifteen years ago, OK?' I am quite shouty too, which is something I worry about … when I'm gone, will my big, throbbing, angry penis-vein in the middle of my forehead be the only thing the kids remember about me? Are they having a nice childhood, or is living with a furious dickhead going to cause them serious psychological harm? What are the trigger points for becoming a criminal mastermind? Very much hope it's not sending a child to their room for effectively telling the truth when outing his parents as the Easter Bunny to a younger sibling, because that absolutely did not happen … Recently, I read an article written by a guy who didn't believe in shouting at his children because he thought it was damaging; instead, he would ask 'what should you have done instead?' Thinking this might be a more nurturing approach to my own disciplinary predicament, the question was posed to my daughter shortly after finding her assaulting her brother with a kids' bible.

'What should you have done, sweetheart?'

'Errr, used the encyclopaedia?'

Righto.

There's also regret about how they both entered the world – the fact I didn't do it 'properly', and guilt that Evelyn doesn't go to ballet on a Saturday because we're always at football with Jack and Steve works weekends. I'm constantly in turmoil about what we allow them to do, and what we don't – for example, they're not allowed to be on the school's social media account, meaning they have to be put in corners when photos are taken and they irrationally hate me for it. We're currently mid-battle with eight-year-old Jack because I refuse point-blank to let him have Fortnite, despite every single one of his friends having it; and apparently wanting to keep him shielded from violence and 50-year-old men pretending to be young boys on the internet makes me a monster. You feel as though you can't do right for doing wrong.

The biggest of all the guilts, however, spawned from something completely out of my – and the rest of the world's – control and was a result of the Covid pandemic. Homeschooling. Once a word reserved for those who didn't want to mainstream educate, it now has the ability to strike fear into the heart of pretty much every parent around the globe. Naturally, the burden of educating our children predominately fell into the hands of women. Come on, lads, have we not done enough?! Apparently not. Surveys showed an overwhelming amount of women being put in the impossible position of trying to balance their professional life with being a full-time mother, teacher, chef, cleaner, personal trainer, receptionist to the Amazon man, and motivational life coach to people who were more concerned about catching Pokémon than the coronavirus. It was almost a reassuring constant to see the gender gap still alive and well during such a dark and uncertain time. My mental health, along with the children's, was absolutely affected by the situation we found ourselves in. There are those who are born to teach, and those who are born to scream silently into a pillow as feral children beat each other with phonics flashcards. The daughter of a retired primary school teacher, I thought I'd be a natural in the home classroom, didn't I? Turns out I was a horrible cross between *Annie*'s Miss Hannigan and *Matilda*'s Miss Trunchbull. My brain was constantly foggy with everything that needed doing, and every day felt like Groundhog Day … Eat, teach, shout, get interrupted on Zoom, put the TV on for the kids and ignore them for five hours, repeat. Women, by nature, are brilliant multitaskers, but sometimes it can be to our detriment – there's an assumption we'll just crack on until we literally crack. Yes, some of us chose to have babies, but that doesn't mean we chose *that* life. The guilt was immeasurable. Conscious of not spending enough time with the kids during the day, but still needing to work, I'd be constantly snapping at them for demanding my attention or not knowing the answer to a maths question I couldn't even work out. Every night there were tears at my failings, and at the prospect the kids were going to grow up thinking Super Mario was a real, and somewhat eccentric, Italian uncle.

Mothers were put in the impossible position of juggling everything, and catching nothing. No one enjoyed homeschooling, not even the kids, who initially thought it was going to be a blast, until they realised Mummy-school was an absolute shit show filled with lots of passive aggressive chat about Daddy being 'out' at work, followed by full-blown arguments when he dared to suggest he'd had a tough day spent with fellow adults not sounding out 's-h-e-d' for the thousandth time. My only hope is that the kids are young enough to forget that pretty awful time in our lives, and that one day I can park the guilt that came with my stab at becoming a teacher – I definitely would have got an Ofsted rating of 'Fuck-Awful'. I do feel as though it's in a mother's DNA to feel guilty about anything and EVERYTHING, but it's probably about time we went easy on ourselves and settled on a fair trial because we're our own worst bloody enemy. Deep down, all our kids really care about is time together, love, Netflix and snacks – never forget the snacks.

Along with all the guilt, there's also an acceptance that I'll worry about my children until my dying day, and probably even after that … I'll be up in heaven (or down in hell, depending), still fretting as to whether (at the age of 60-odd) they've wiped their bums properly, have been to the doctor about that lingering cough, and have nutritionally offset eating a whole bag of Haribo by following it with an apple. I'm terrified about leaving this world – and them – behind. The thought of never seeing their faces again sends me into the biggest emotional downwards spiral. My biggest fear, however, is living in a world where they don't exist. Prior to having kids, I never really understood it when people would say they'd lay down their lives for someone. Now I get it. I'd happily give my life to save theirs, because without them my life would cease to exist anyway.

At present, our current daily battles revolve around shoes, not using listening ears, and their refusal to eat anything green unless it's come out of their noses … but bigger problems loom in the not-too-distant future, in the form of the teenage years. By that point, I'll be a total MILF (Massively Interfering Lunatic Female) who's desperate to know every aspect of their lives, along with their exact whereabouts at all times of the day and night. Right now, I'm not sure who I'm worried about the most … Jack, in case he takes his Mario Kart lockdown learnings into the real word and onto real roads, or Evelyn, in a nightclub toilet getting punched in the face for telling another girl how much cuter her own vagina is. Do we think it's OK to keep them locked up in the house forever? No? Frowned upon, probably. The prospect of social media also scares the shit out of me. As someone who has seen both the light and dark of the internet, I'd like to keep them both away from it for as long as humanly possible, but I can already foresee the double-standard arguments heading my way due to my highly ironical choice of career. 'DO AS I SAY, NOT AS I DO!' Worry, along with so many other aspects, is just another part of the job description no one really told you about, along with how batshit crazy kids go when you accuse them of being tired, or their weird attachments to inanimate objects – we once had a very unfortunate incident after I'd been on a hen party and one of them found a penis straw they refused to let out of their sight.

Now my kids are a bit older, and I'm finally out of the hazy baby and toddler years, I'm stuck with a bit of a conundrum … Am I done? Do I want any more? Now, this may seem like madness if you've actually stuck it out through all the chapters and have found yourself at this concluding part. I'M OUT! Why would I put myself back through some of the hardest years all over again? I pretty much get a full night's sleep, they're both in full-time education (Covid depending), and I can finally leave the house with a relatively small handbag again. Life is undeniably easier. But … there's an ache … On seeing a fresh-out-the-oven baby, complete with new-vag smell, my ovaries start to throb. As it happens, I'm actually on a baby ban … already got two points on my licence and Steve really doesn't want me to get a third. He's very much a 'two's company, three's a crowd' kind of guy – although I can't help but feel his attitude might change if ever I suggested a threesome … Here's the thing, though – I don't know whether it's a genuine want or if it's my body tricking me into thinking we need to continually populate the human race. The only person I know who is 'fully' done is one of my friends who had two kids, went for a third and ended up with twins. Not even a shirtless Chris Hemsworth, holding the world's cutest baby, Thor cape fluttering behind and with come-to-bed 'it's hammer time' eyes, could change her mind. Now, if placed in a similar scenario, I'd more than likely drop my knickers faster than lightning, before he changed his mind and said 'can't touch this'. What to do, though, if you think you want another baby, but your partner doesn't? If my future happiness depended on it, he'd eventually cave and take one for the team … but I'd feel shitty about putting him in that situation. Also, in the aftermath of the miscarriage of what would have been our third child, there was a huge part of me that immediately shut down the prospect of adding to our brood. At the time, to me, it was a sign things weren't meant to be … an omen. Given how absolutely awful it was, there was no way I could put myself, or anyone I loved, through that torment again. Time, however, is a healer, and eventually physical and mental scars begin to fade – bringing with them fresh perspectives and questions. Retrospectively, I had pretty awful PTSD after Jack was born, but at the time didn't recognise it, assuming it was normal and probably how most new mums felt after the shock of childbirth. Making the decision to have Evelyn, although difficult in the sense of having to push myself through a mental barrier (and poor Steve had to deal with me crying every time we attempted baby-making sex), was almost easier in a way because I didn't want Jack to be an only child – I'd just have to get over it, and under it. This time round, with one of each – both happy and healthy – why rock the boat? Maybe it's hormones, maybe I'm longing to replace what was lost, maybe I actually want one … who knows? Clearly not me.

What I've discovered about my own arrival into adult life is that it has mostly revolved around preparing small people for theirs. Yes, sometimes there's a desire to be a free spirit who's able to drop life at a minute's notice in order to go have it large in Ibiza, getting pissed on two gin and tonics and living my best life. Apart from … I wouldn't really, because that would mean not having my little family and that would be shit. I can't imagine not seeing my handsome Jack's breath-taking blue eyes, or hearing his infectious little laugh … same goes for listening to Evelyn singing songs at the top of her lungs day in, day out (in an American accent because I let her watch too much Netflix), and finding her handwritten notes under my pillow saying how much she loves me.

Granted, my twenties were an amazing, hedonistic, and carefree existence, but I'm now at a point of thinking 'thank God I don't have to do that again' – mainly because it was the early noughties and kitten heels with combat trousers were all the rage. Horrific. Looking at myself now, as a proper grown-up, do I have all my shit together? No. Probably not. I'm still always pathologically late for everything, wine continues to makes me hurl, and I never did crack my nine times table. Deep down, am I still the same girl who was in search of a life less ordinary, keen to get as many items ticked off the pre-kids 'Bucket-Fanny List' as possible? Absolutely not. I reckon I'm better.

Although I feel very strongly about motherhood not defining me, it's definitely changed me. My wild ride into parenthood has evolved me into someone who's stronger, wiser, funnier, and fiercer than I could have ever imagined being, and, more importantly, I'm not 'just a mum' … I'm Jack and Evelyn's mum – a practical, decisive, danger-spotting, somewhat aggressive meerkat with a killer gut instinct and a fur-covered C-section shelf, and do you know what? I wouldn't change it for the motherfucking world.

Acknowledgements

OK, thank you time! Just a warning, I might end up going a little Gwyneth Paltrow on you here … not in the sense of trying to flog anyone a vagina candle, more her Oscar speech.

So I should probably start with my two beautiful babies – who hate me calling them 'babies' – but once they've read this and discovered the literal ins and outs of how they were conceived, they're going to have a bigger axe to grind … So, to my babies – without you none of this would be possible – when you first came into my life, I had no idea you'd be the absolute making of me in so many ways. You opened my heart, mind, creativity – and abdominal wall. Thank you for coming on so much of this journey with me, and for making my dreams of being a Mummy and an author come true. I LOVE YOU SO MUCH and even as I'm writing this, in the dead of night, I've just snuck into your rooms and had a little sob at how utterly perfect you are in every single way. Mummy will never stop doing that, just a heads up to your future partners – it's going to get weird. I'm so sorry that I haven't been as much of a 'fun mum' as I should have been during the process of creating this book – I promise I'll make it up to you. Hopefully you had a great time with Daddy, Uncle Mario and Auntie Princess Peach while I was typing away upstairs. My foundations, inspirations, and motivations – you amaze me every single day and I'm so incredibly lucky to have you both in my life. NEVER stop being your wonderful, beautiful, silly-sausage selves.

Steve, thank you for being my ride or die, and for your sperm. The most handsome man I've ever met – who'd have thought that an encounter in a nightclub called Evolution alllllllll those years ago would result in everything we have today? From day dot, you've known and supported my ambition to hide from you all and create something not only for myself – but for others. Never batting an eyelid at all the daft things I do, even on coming home to find me painted bright blue, in a giant headlouse costume, or honing my rapping skills – you might not be Dwayne Johnson, but you're my absolute rock. You've never stood in my way, or tried to diminish my shine and for that, along with letting me put your lockdown haircut video on the internet, I am forever grateful. You spur me on to work harder (by not laughing at my jokes) and are quite possibly the best beaver a girl could ever wish for. Thanks for always putting the bin out. I love you more than I probably tell you.

To my parents – cheers for also embarking on 'grumpy pumpy' and creating me! Legends. Dad, I get my funny from you (and sadly, my knees); Mum your other 50% has enabled me to string those comic musings into legible sentences that have now been published for the world to read. MADNESS. Thank you both for believing in me, and for being incredibly proud of everything I've done – apart from that time I drove into a stationary double decker bus, the neighbour's car and your gatepost (twice) in Mum's Rover. A published author! Who'd have thought?! All those years of screaming at me to do my homework, while I ignored you, have finally paid off! Shout out to my big sister too, for giving me my first and in-depth insight into the sometimes-physical art of sibling rivalry. Sorry I once threw a Swingball bat at your face.

My literary agent, Lauren, thank you so much for sliding into my DMs and propositioning me in the best way possible. You gave me the confidence to believe that other people might be interested in what I had to say, the patience to sit through those sketchy first drafts and my regular wobbles of self-doubt.

LUCY!! My Momager! A great friend who came back into my life at just the right time. Destiny, right? Book world was something I threw you into, and you've been such a great support – who else could I WhatsApp voice message 300 times a day? The kids hear 'Agent Lucy's' voice about as often as they hear my own. Here's to many more research trips and cannonballing into pretentious swimming pools.

To Gen and the whole team at HarperNorth, I'm so humbled you decided to take a risk on this Scouse mum of two. Your wisdom, experience, and professionalism when faced with various urban dictionary synonyms for 'muffs' continues to astound me. Your vision for me as an author has never wavered, and I hope I do you all proud.

Last, but by no means least, to everyone who has chosen to follow me over the years (on social media, not from behind bushes) … THANK YOU! Without you taking the time to comment on my content, or share it with friends and family, there would be no *Tired & Tested*. I see you all as friends that I've just not got drunk with yet, and I hope the feeling is mutual. You're all bloody amazing!

Harper
North

Book Credits

HarperNorth would like to thank the following staff and contributors for their involvement in making this book a reality:

Hannah Avery
Fionnuala Barrett
Claire Boal
Charlotte Brown
Sarah Burke
Alan Cracknell
Jonathan de Peyer
Anna Derkacz
Tom Dunstan
Kate Elton
Mick Fawcett
Monica Green
CJ Harter
Graham Holmes
Megan Jones
Jean-Marie Kelly
Oliver Malcolm
Alice Murphy-Pyle
Adam Murray
Holly Ovenden
Genevieve Pegg
Rob Pinney
Agnes Rigou
Florence Shepherd
Angela Snowden
Emma Sullivan
Katrina Troy